Meridian Massage is not only the quintessential must-read for anyone looking *Chinese Medicine and Cindy's innovative hands-on approach, but also for thos̄* *'something more.' Cindy delivers a deep, insightful and remarkably down-to-earth approach to teaching this riʼ̄* *material.*

Meridian Massage lays a solid foundation while simultaneously inspiring the reader to achieve an understanding of Qi, Nature, the ways of the Universe and how to tap into the innate healing energy within each of us. The vast amount of substance conveyed with the turn of every page, intertwines love, understanding, awareness, and peace into the tapestry of Chinese Medicine. This is an invigorating way to embark on your healing journey, or to simply strengthen your roots as you navigate along your path.

As a licensed Acupuncture Physician myself, it is refreshing to find an approach that truly encompasses the mind, body, emotions and spirit. I only wish I could have experienced this book when beginning my exploration of Oriental Medicine. If you are searching for a simple yet profound technique to heal yourself, your family, or your clients, you have discovered it! Cindy offers guidance and instruction that emanate warmth, enthusiasm and brilliance.

Jessica Cudar, DOM, AP
Acupuncture Physician

Cindy Black has accomplished the impressive task of distilling the fundamentals from the vast system of traditional Chinese medicine, and creating a clearly descriptive and beautifully illustrated book. Due to her experience as a Licensed Acupuncturist, she is adept at explaining this ancient system and its practical uses for all hands-on therapists. As a professional bodyworker and instructor, I consider this book a valuable asset for myself, my students, and my clients. It serves as an accessible entryway to understanding our energetic anatomy and its significant relationship to our health.

In the classroom, Cindy displays an unusual talent of clear presentation combined with sharp wit and humor, which consistently makes learning a pleasure by bringing her material alive. That she has also accomplished this task with her book is another testament to her expertise. Her book is perfect for massage therapists and other hands-on healers. I would also highly recommend it to anyone who wants to know more about the ancient art of Chinese medicine and their own remarkable, potent energy for healing.

Bernadette Fiocca, LMT (Private Practice since 1984)
Shiatsu and Energy Palpation Instructor at Finger Lakes School of Massage, Ithaca, NY.

Great bodyworkers find the midpoint between their clients' energy and their own, and work from that space. They are able to strip away who they think they are, what they feel they need to do, and whom they think the person on their table is, in order to be guided from that harmonious place.

Meridian Massage: Opening Pathways to Vitality is not just a valuable instruction manual, resource, or reference book. Rather, unlike other books of its nature, it also affords guidance to the practitioner about how to access the Qi of the meridians. She encourages us to do the necessary inner work to cultivate our own Qi, in order to tap into the spirit of the points without the use of needles.

This book is filled with depth and reverence for an ancient art, interwoven with the wisdom of the Tao. It offers a fresh perspective which is refreshing and sometimes humorous, never dry and rote. Descriptions are vivid, stories are poignant, her writing is engaging, and her passion is evident. In a way that is easily digestible, Cindy has made available to modern practitioners a buffet to savor.

Teresa L. Crosier, D.O.M., Dipl. C.M., Dipl. Ac., author of *In Harmony With Nature*
Owner, Combining Cultures Acupuncture & Herbal Clinic in Albuquerque, NM
Associate Professor at Southwest Acupuncture College in Santa Fe, NM

Meridian Massage
Opening Pathways to Vitality

Cindy Black

To Andrea,

for a lifetime of love and adventure

Dedication

To all of my teachers, known and unknown
To all of my students, known and unknown
Thank you for sharing the path with me

In Memory

of my Mother, Sally Barker

Acknowledgements

My gratitude to Paul Cash for his wise editing and ability to formulate my thoughts into a real book.

Jessica Joswiak spent endless hours getting every meridian and point picture just right.

Andrea Barras designed the beautiful book in your hands.

A few years ago, four special people took a chance and enrolled in my first Meridian Massage Certification Program. Their enthusiasm and trust laid the foundation for this book: Paula Begel, Sue Bissell, Carol Horton, Janet Klock, thank you from the depths of my heart.

Fortunately, I crossed paths with Khadro, who revealed the heart and soul of Chinese medicine to me.

My deepest appreciation to Edie Pett, Christina Polnyj- Pollman, Curt Pollman, Annie Powell, Peris Gumz, Teresa Crosier, William Horden, Linda Ruth, Lori Yelensky and Kc Rossi for believing in me all these years.

ISBN: 978-0-9969718-1-2

24 23 22 21 20 19 18 17 16
10 9 8 7 6 5 4 3 2 1

Table of Contents

Introduction

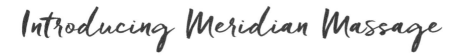

Introducing Meridian Massage

Health and happiness are results of abundant, flowing, harmonious Qi. Meridian Massage offers hands-on assistance to move, nourish, and feel Qi. It is that simple.

Simple is so far from easy that it takes a whole book to explain the principles of this work and how to put them into practice. It has taken me thirty years to get simple. I hope to help you get simple sooner.

Components of Meridian Massage

Meridian Massage has seven components:

1. Anatomy
2. Classical Chinese medical theory
3. Western massage techniques
4. Chinese massage techniques
5. A relationship with Nature
6. Self-awareness
7. Practicing ourselves what we ask our clients to practice

As hands-on practitioners, we receive direct experience of the client's body through our hands and kinesthetic sense. Blending that with our detailed intellectual knowledge of human anatomy and the meridian system, we weave our impressions and sensations into a treatment that supports Qi toward circulation and harmonization.

To be "holistic" means to include everything, all parts of the whole. Holistic health is supposed to include body, mind, and spirit. The practice of Meridian Massage takes this premise literally.

Holistic healing is a huge undertaking. Nothing less than attending fully to body, mind, and spirit will result in healing signified by fundamental changes in the body, mind, and spirit.

Meridian Massage draws from the ancient tradition of Classical Chinese medicine and applies it in the context of our modern Western world. We combine elements of Classical Chinese medical theory, Western massage technique, and Chinese massage technique. Embodying the practices and theories involved takes perseverance, curiosity, patience, dedication, and compassion in order to develop an inner knowing and sensitivity that guides the practice. We must develop an intimate relationship with Nature around us, our inner nature, and the ability to practice ourselves what we tell our clients to do.

Because of these requirements, we practitioners have as much to gain from the study of Meridian Massage as our clients do in receiving it. We can only give that which we actually have within ourselves to give. If you seek to give healing and love to others, you must have healing and love within yourself to give.

The process of learning Meridian Massage contains within it ways of connecting to your own self-love, healing, and wisdom. By going through this process yourself, you will be able to transmit your healing wisdom to others.

Going Within

Every great wisdom tradition calls us to go within to find our answers, to listen to our hearts, to know the One, God, Source, Divine. It follows that every great healing tradition would support that pathway toward wholeness. In the ancient roots of Classical Chinese medicine, in Taoism, we find this directive as the foundation to healing.

To feel Qi, to feel ourselves, to gain access to the wisdom of our experiences, we must turn our attention inward.

"The Tao that can be told is not the eternal Tao." [1] *This is the famous first line of the Taoist classic the Tao Te Ching. It can also be translated as, "The way that can be explained is not the eternal Way" or "The path that is well marked is not the eternal Path." Although the true Way or Path has always existed in eternity and rigorously conforms to precise laws, it must always be discovered for oneself. The ordinary isolated intellect is not the agent through which the living, present moment can be experienced.* [2]

Turning the attention inward and connecting with our wordless nature is challenging yet possible. Once we are able to identify and follow the path inward, we benefit from bountiful internal resources. As we practice ways of keeping these resources flowing, we experience increased physical vitality, mental clarity, and the wise guidance of our Spirit. Meridian Massage is a holistic healing approach and a path of personal growth.

What Is Meridian Massage?

I use this term as it is generic, describing a general practice of massage based on the meridians of Chinese medicine. Meridian Massage is not so much a specific technique as a specific holistic approach to massage based on principles of Classical Chinese medicine.

Fundamental to Chinese medicine is Qi ("chee"). Qi is that which enlivens us. Living entities move. The "thing" that is present in a body we call "alive" and is gone in a body that we pronounce "dead" is Qi. Our body, mind, and spirit all depend on Qi. The quantity, quality, and flow of our Qi results in our state of health.

Qi does not circulate because someone prompts it to, Qi circulates because that is the nature of Qi. Qi moves, flows, changes, appears, and recedes in cycles of time and space beyond human understanding. It also circulates in rhythms accessible to human understanding—the planetary rotation around the Sun, the seasons, the cycles of the Moon, the passing of a day, the waxing and waning of a human life.

If Qi does not require human intervention in order to move, in order to "Be," then what good can we do as Meridian Massage practitioners? The Qi of one person can support the harmony of Qi within another person. We all have the direct experience of Qi being stuck or out of harmony—this is known as pain or illness. Yes, our innate physiology and Qi are always working their way back to homeostasis, balance, and flow. But sometimes, to regain our balance, we need the help of another person.

The good that a healer can do is to support this return to balance in another. The healer must always be aware of being a participant in a greater process, not the holder of the process.

Meridian Massage is based fully in the belief that we are part of something greater than ourselves, that as practitioners we participate in this greater wisdom. Qi flows in the meridians, as you will see diagrammed throughout this book. We offer massage to benefit the flow of Qi already in process within our clients. We are in service to the bigger picture that we know exists yet cannot fully comprehend or control. We follow our intuition as we discover precise anatomical locations for the best improvisation of contact that will allow the Qi of this particular person at this particular time to regain balance.

Meridian Massage can be utilized by any hands-on practitioner in any environment from sports massage to chakra clearing, NMT, or medical massage. Making simple contact with Qi in the meridians has supported people for thousands of years. The effectiveness of this simple method is rooted in combining detailed anatomical understanding of the meridians and acupoint locations with the sensitivity of the practitioner.

Meeting Points

The goal of Meridian Massage is to facilitate the meeting, communication, and peaceful relationship between Yin and Yang within a human being. In Western terms, this is the meeting of the left brain and right brain, masculine and feminine, conscious and unconscious, body and mind. There are countless possible meeting points in our inner worlds.

The ability to flow easily between our creative, broad, systemic right-brain thinking and our linear, focused left-brain thinking offers real possibilities for figuring out how to live the true potentials of our life. When we can shift from our directed, ambitious, and active masculine energy to our receptive, co-creative, and reflective feminine energy as easily as we choose between coffee and tea, we have found real freedom of choice.

When our inner world is one of peace and harmony, we set the stage for our physical, emotional, and mental health. For there to be peace and harmony, there must be communication. A meeting point is a place where left and right, conscious and unconscious, body and energy, "good" and "bad" literally face one another to mediate their differences in service to the "greater good."

Yin from the Earth combined with Yang of the Sky creates an individual who is a unique expression of these two primary forces. Each one of us is a singular container of Yin and Yang, of two parts or energies. This primary duality shows up everywhere as conscious and unconscious, mind and body, energy and matter, sympathetic and parasympathetic nervous system, activity and stillness, inner life and outer life.

It looks like we are a single unit but we can feel that we are not. "One part of me wants this, the other part wants that." "My mind says go but my heart says stay."

We learn from our family, friends, society, schools, media, and culture how to navigate amidst these forces. The course of that learning includes judging some as good and some as bad. Bad becomes hidden from ourselves as we leave it behind in order to be good, according to the environment around us. In that process we learn an inner process of disconnecting, walling off, moving away from impulses and parts of ourselves that are "bad" or "not useful." This process creates a division and separation between Yin and Yang, body and mind, conscious and unconscious, etc.

When the internal energies are separated from one another, they do not communicate and thus cannot benefit from one another, cannot nourish, invigorate, protect, or inspire one another. For individuals, our inner lives become smaller, more tense and strained as we try to maintain the narrow path that we think we must live in order to be good, right, successful. This strain limits us physically, mentally, emotionally, and spiritually.

Physically, our organs will suffer and over time we will have to contend with various ailments related to this or that organ's dysfunction. Mentally we suffer with confusion, lack of focus. Emotionally we suffer with shame, frustration, fear, anxiety, sadness. Spiritually we suffer lack of hope, inspiration, possibility, or faith.

Classical Chinese medicine is holistic. Infused with the spiritual traditions of Taoism and Buddhism, created through observation of Nature, reverence for Nature, and a sense of interrelation with the Universe, it offers a clear path of return to wholeness. In this form of medicine, Organs hold, transform, and communicate energy (Qi). The continuum from Spirit to Organ is a web of meridians where the Qi, the information, flows and expresses itself as thought, emotion, physical form and function, mind, and spirit.

Meridian Massage relies on the path of Chinese medicine to facilitate each person's re-weaving of their inner world at various meeting points. Meeting points are not physical locations. Meeting points are sensed internally when we are able to feel our breath, to literally feel our organs and receive their stories, memories, wisdom. When we at last turn toward our shadow and allow ourselves to hear its story, we are meeting ourselves. Dropping defenses, removing walls, letting energy flow again, this is the process of harmonizing Qi, of opening the meridians to allow for Yin and Yang to communicate, to flow, to balance.

Chinese medicine promises that when the Qi is plentiful and flowing, so are our physical body, mind, and spirit. Meridian Massage facilitates this process using hands-on techniques.

Human Spirit as Medicine

Hands-on medicine or healing is only as "good" or "potent" as is the owner of those hands. This is why receiving massage from different massage therapists feels so different. Why is it that the same style of massage given to the same area of the body feels so different and provides different results? Because the inner state of the therapists is different.

Each practitioner is a person with an inner world. The relative balance and harmony within the practitioner has the greatest impact on their hands-on work. This inner harmony (or disharmony) has a bigger impact than the types of massage they have learned, the degrees they possess, or the years they have been practicing.

Because our state of harmony is the key factor in our work, Meridian Massage requires inner development for its success.

The Practitioner Is Actually the Medicine

Medicine that can be healing can also cause harm. Humans have the potential for both. We are endowed with an extraordinary brain coupled with hands that are the most dexterous of all creatures on a physically upright frame. From this combination, human technology has given birth to beautiful cultures and civilizations, and has done terrible harm to ourselves and other creatures. We have all harmed others and ourselves, we have all benefited others and ourselves.

In the field of medicine, all practitioners know that their work can heal or harm. A surgeon's knife can harm or heal. The physician's pharmaceuticals and the herbalist's herbs can harm or heal. Our hands can harm or heal. The difference depends on the practitioner.

Hands-on practitioners dedicate themselves to self-development in order to become the most potent and beneficial medicine they can be. We know that with certain medications we must "shake well before use." Meridian Massage practitioners must be "integrated well" before use.

When we know how to shift from Yin to Yang within ourselves, we are able to modify ourselves moment to moment in order to facilitate the processes of inner work our client is engaging in. We learn how to offer the "correct dose of ourselves" as modifications in our speech, amount of pressure, where we touch, how we touch, our questions, suggestions, and silence.

We will always be in process with this integration. As we practice ourselves we gain insights from our unconscious mind, our Organs, cells, Qi, and our connection to Nature. These insights, integrated within our inner world, become the unique expression of our personal hands-on medicine.

There are three key principles to keep always in mind while we work at this integration:

> *As practitioners, we enter into a larger process of healing in partnership with our clients, who remain in charge of their journey toward harmony and health.*

Tempting as it may be to think that we can heal another person, the reality is quite different. Yes, we can understand a great deal about anatomy, physiology, pathology, Qi, and Nature. We can know more about these specializations than our client does. But we can never know more about our clients than the clients know about themselves.

We can open doors, but it is they who must take it upon themselves to move through the openings toward balance, peace, and health. We can support their immune system, their Qi, their Organs—but it is their immune system, their Qi, their Organs that complete the actual healing. Even pharmaceutical medicines can only enhance or interrupt the inherent processes of physiology—no medicine can create a process that is not native to the body.

If a surgeon removes a tumor, it is the body that ultimately heals the wound and readjusts itself to a structure without that tumor. The removal of a tumor does not remove the physiology that created the tumor, nor does it prevent that physiology from creating another tumor. The surgeon can celebrate the removal as a heroic healing endeavor, but the ground that created it will be the ultimate judge of success or lack of it. The stamina, the intelligence, the regenerative nature of the body-mind-spirit is itself the only "thing" that can do the invisible true work of returning to energetic harmony that will manifest as physical, mental, and emotional health.

If we as practitioners keep our mind and heart on this reality, we will find ourselves in partnership with a healing force much greater and beneficial than what we can offer from just ourselves as individuals. Working in this way is quieter and less glamorous than proclaiming ourselves the origin of healing. From this point of view, we are in partnership with something we cannot fully comprehend, control, or call our own. I call this being of service to others through being in service to a compassionate intelligence that is the Source of all life.

Developing this relationship to Nature or Source is available to everyone. As such, it is a practice that does not allow any one person to claim its power as their own. It offers us a path for our own well-being as well as a path of service to others, so that they may find relief from their suffering as this healing energy guides their body-mind-spirit toward harmony and balance. After coming to this balance, our clients may very well pursue their own relationship with this bigger energy in order to maintain their health without the need of our services. This would be the best outcome.

> *Our central effort is to be in communion with our own Qi. Our actions spring from this connection as we allow our work to be guided by the wisdom of Qi.*

We are living in these bodies for a relatively short time. We may have spent two years, or even thirty years studying and practicing. These are tiny increments of time compared to the infinite time of the Source Qi, the Mysterious Source of Nature, the Tao.

Think of the Undifferentiated Source Qi, the Tao, as the Sun and your own Qi as a ray of that Sun. The method of connecting with that vast intelligence is to follow your ray of energy, your Qi, back to that of the Undifferentiated Source Qi. Allow the Source Qi to guide your actions during the treatment and your work will be more effective and valuable to your client.

Inner work is required to know your own Qi, to balance your Yin and Yang, to feel your connection to Nature, to know your connection to Source Qi.

> *Although the present moment may not make logical sense to us, we trust the flow of the One-Source which ultimately provides the resolution of imbalance and the return to well-being.*

Our five senses are very good at measuring, noticing, locating physical manifestations at any moment in time. Just as an X-ray can take a picture of a bone at a certain time, our senses meet a physically manifested person at a moment in time.

If we consider this moment in time that we are sensing another person as the total picture, we would be as incorrect in our assessment as an X-ray that declares that the break in the bone it shows is the whole story. We know that an X-ray can show us a broken bone, and we also know that for years previous that bone was fully intact. And we know from our experience that it is already beginning to heal and will heal completely in time.

Just like the X-ray, our five senses interpret a physical reality rather than the energy that created the physical reality. We can see a five-hundred-year-old redwood tree, but we cannot see the seed that began the story. We can learn to use an ability beyond the five senses to bring our mind back to that seed, which will inevitably bring us back to the tree from which that seed fell. We find ourselves lost in a stream of incomprehensible manifestations—beyond the reach of anything logically understandable.

What can be sensed is a rhythm of manifestations: seed, sprout, tree, seed, sprout, tree. These manifestations arise from undifferentiated energy that is beyond our five senses. Energy has its own logic of processes and unfolding. Energy sprouts many different manifestations that may seem illogical when viewed only from within the confines of our five senses. But seen from the point view of energy, it can all make sense.

How can two different points of view of the same phenomena be true at the same time? Think of our solar system. When the Sun is viewed from Earth, it appears that the Earth is still and the Sun is moving. But when we view the solar system as a whole, we see that the Sun is still and the Earth is spinning and rotating around the Sun. Both views are true as seen through the lenses of the five senses—it is only that other ability beyond our five senses that can hold the reality of these two seemingly opposing truths and remain peaceful.

Imagine we are witnessing the decline and death of another. Our five senses can pick up the changes in physical manifestation of the person before us. We can reach out and try to alleviate the physical suffering, but we know that we cannot stop the process of death unfolding before our eyes. This suffering makes no logical sense. But from the point of view of the unseen energetic Soul-Spirit of this person, it is the shedding of a physical body in preparation for its next stage in the cycle of Energetics that is beyond our five senses.

If we view only the physical journey at this point, we will suffer as we observe and feel the suffering of another. If we view only the energetic journey, we may be so detached that we cannot offer solace. It is only by finding a way, through constant practice, to hold both realities within us, that we can offer solace and hope to another while we ourselves remain peaceful and hopeful within.

Death heightens our awareness of this duality, but the duality is true every moment. It is true every time we assess another person. Our presence will be one of peace, harmony, hope, and healing if we can maintain this level of understanding in every interaction with every person.

How to Use This Book

This book has five parts.

Part 1: Theory - Principles of Meridian Massage introduces you to foundational concepts of Classical Chinese medicine: the relationship of Nature and human life, Qi, Yin, Yang, the substances of human life, the Five Elements and the Organ Systems. It lays the foundation for the practices of Meridian Massage.

In Part 2: Tools of the Trade, we dive into the twelve meridians, which are the pathways where Qi flows in the body. We consider the nature of each meridian within the framework of the theory in Part 1. I discuss in detail points commonly used in hands-on practice, giving you the point's location, tips for locating the point, and information about the use of each point.

From Part 3: Hands-on Meridian Massage, you will learn how to utilize meridians and points within your practice of massage to support health and vitality.

From Part 4: Common Conditions - The Meridian Massage Approach to Common Conditions Encountered in a Hands-on Healing Practice, you will learn how to consider common Western ailments from the perspective of Meridian Massage.

From Part 5: Living Principles - Caring for Yourself to Care for Others, you will learn how to continue cultivating your own practice of moving and harmonizing your Qi in order to continue your learning and maintain your health.

Part 1

Theory: Principles of Meridian Massage

1: Introduction to Chinese Medicine

The Tao that can be told is not the eternal Tao.
The name that can be named is not the eternal name.
The nameless is the beginning of heaven and earth.
The named is the mother of ten thousand things.
Ever desireless, one can see the mystery.
Ever desiring, one can see the manifestations.
These two spring from the same source but differ in name;
This appears as darkness.
Darkness within darkness.
The gate to all mystery. [3]

The basic principles of Meridian Massage derive from Classical Chinese medicine, which sees us within the context of our environment. Classical Chinese medicine grew out of Taoism, which was the prevailing philosophy and spirituality in ancient China. This provided the context for the development of the medicine. "Classical Chinese medicine" is a modern term used to describe Chinese medicine that draws upon the Taoist roots. "Traditional Chinese medicine" generally does not include the principles of Taoist philosophy within its practices.

We are a part of Nature, Nature is a part of us. Nature, the Universe, and all beings are in relationship with one another: Earth always below us, the vast sky above, the Sun, the Moon, the planets and stars even further away. We are understood as being in relationship to the elements of Nature around us. And these same elements of Nature are understood to be within us.

Observing ourselves in this way, we can get closer to the notion that a human being is a microcosmic representation of the larger Universe. We have seasons of birth, growth, adulthood, decline, and death just as a tree is subject to Spring, Summer, Late Summer, Fall, and Winter. We are made of the same material that makes everything in the world around us. To know ourselves, we look to Nature as the mirror of what we humans might actually be.

What we can see, touch, feel, hear, and taste are known as physical manifestations. Manifestations from what basis?

When we see a tree, we see only a part of it. The roots are hidden beneath the surface of the ground. The seed from which the tree originally sprouted is completely gone. In a similar way, a physical manifestation grows out of energy that is not perceived by our five senses. This original, vast, mysterious Source from which everything came is a Mystery.

"The nameless is the beginning of heaven and earth," [4] declares the Tao Te Ching.

Every manifestation, every thing, person, plant, and bug originates from this vast and nameless Mystery. The energy of this Mystery is eternal. Each of us has a spark of this energy within us. This spark of life will return to its Mysterious Source when the physical manifestation within which it resides comes to an end.

In Western science we find a similar revelation that humans are composed of "star dust." The molecules that make up the stars are the same as the molecules that form our bodies. As Carl Sagan wrote, "The nitrogen in our DNA, the calcium in our teeth, the iron in our blood, the carbon in our apple pies were made in the interiors of collapsing stars. We are made of starstuff." [5] Some of the material in our bodies is from the very beginning of the Universe.

Living in Nature

Nature has cycles, temperatures, weather, an ecology of plants, animals, and elements that depend on each other for life. When we look to Chinese medicine for direction on how to live, it points us toward Nature. Although humans have created living conditions that protect us from many of the forces of Nature, we are still part of the bigger system within which we live.

If we can live in harmony with the cycles of Nature, it is said, then we will enjoy a healthier, longer, and happier life.

In ancient times, people lived simply. They hunted, fished and were with nature all day. When the weather cooled, they became active to fend off the cold. When the weather heated up in summer, they retreated to cool places. Internally, their emotions were calm and peaceful, and they were without excessive desires. Externally, they did not have the stress of today. They lived without greed and desire, close to nature. They maintained jing shen nei suo, or inner peace and concentration of the mind and spirit. This prevented the pathogens from invading. Therefore, they did not need herbs to treat their internal state, nor did they need acupuncture to treat the exterior. When they did contract disease they simply guided properly the emotions and spirit and redirected the energy flow, using the method of zhu you (prayer, ceremony, shamanism) to heal the condition.

—Yellow Emperor's Classic Medicine [6]

How Do We Bring the Wisdom of Nature into Our Healing?

The ordinary isolated intellect is not the agent through which the living present moment can be experienced. [7]

What are the origins of the manifestations around us? Where did our house, our body, that tree come from? We identify these things with our five senses. Even though we know that our single body is made up of billions of invisible cells, our senses identify a single, formed, manifestation.

Taking this even further, the cells of our body are made up of molecules. Molecules are made up of atoms. Atoms are made up of other miniscule particles, and on and on it goes. Today, even Western science recognizes that these atoms, these "building blocks," are essentially energy. What appears as form, as solid, is actually "made" from energy.

From the Chinese medical perspective, we speak of the formed and the formless, the manifested and the undifferentiated, energy and substance, Yang and Yin. The source of all manifestation is undifferentiated energetic Mystery. This means that all the planets, animals, bugs, and people are from this same common source. The manifestation of this Undifferentiated Source is everything that we can see, hear, touch, taste, smell, feel, name.

Yin and Yang

The dynamism of Yin and Yang is a fundamental principle of Chinese medicine. It applies to the manifested yet ever changing world we live in. When we attend only to what is manifested, we experience things such as cold and hot, moving or still, inside and outside, day and night, hard or soft, left and right. We know this thing in reference to that thing. I know my left because I know where my right is.

This type of perspective is known as duality. We contrast two things such as day and night. Could you know what day is if you did not know night? Can you even describe day without contrasting it with night?

It is simpler to know these contrasting pairs than it is to know or sense the undifferentiated single source from which they emerged. If we can't or won't extend our knowing beyond the manifestations that we can easily sense, we simply get lost in manifestations. We may get attached to manifestations and suffer greatly when they change or end.

This symbol is called Taiji:

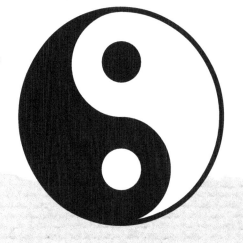

It shows Yin (dark) and Yang (light) flowing within a circle.

A few important details:

- The circle symbolizes the One from which Yin and Yang emerge.

- There is a tiny bit of Yang in the Yin, and of Yin in Yang. This reminds us that nothing is purely one or other. Everything is known in relation to something else.

- The curves remind us that these two forces are always in motion, always dancing with each other.

- From a single thing, from the One, springs two opposing, dependent forces, Yin and Yang.

From these two, everything known emerges and is understood as a particular mixture and manifestation of Yin and Yang.

The Tao that can be told is not the eternal Tao.

The name that can be named is not the eternal name.

The nameless is the beginning of heaven and earth.

The named is the mother of ten thousand things. . . .

Ever desireless, one can see the mystery.

Ever desiring, one can see the manifestations.

These two spring from the same source [One] but differ in name;

This appears as darkness.

Darkness within darkness.

The gate to all mystery. [8]

Although each is a single term, Yin and Yang both encompass many qualities:

YIN	YANG	YIN	YANG
Dark	Bright	Soft	Hard
Cool	Warm	Water	Fire
Damp	Dry	Earth	Sky
Inside	Outside	Moon	Sun
Down	Up	Blood	Qi (energy)
Nighttime	Daytime	Dense	Light
Still	Moving	Material	Immaterial
Receptive	Expressive	Quiet	Loud
Female	Male	Low	High

Imagine it is the middle of a sunny day in summer. What is it like? What is going on? What are people, birds, and animals doing? What does the sky look like? Read the list of Yang qualities again and get a feel for Yang.

Imagine the middle of the night on that same day. What is it like, what is going on, what are people birds animals doing, what does the sky look like? Read the list of Yin qualities again and get a feel for Yin.

The philosophy of Yin and Yang was created by people who lived thousands of years ago. They lived outside, in the elements. They observed nature in order to understand life. You and I have the same opportunity to observe nature in order to embody an understanding of Yin and Yang. It is as simple as noticing what is different in everything you can observe during the day and during the night.

Each thing, person, or event can be understood as a blend of Yin and Yang. The nature or qualities of the thing, person, or event are revealed by the relative amounts of Yin and Yang.

For example, some people have loud voices, are always moving even when seated, and look forward to their fast-paced daily group aerobic class with loud music. Other people have quiet voices, tend toward stillness, and look forward to their daily practice of meditation, in silence, by themselves.

These descriptions are stereotypical to highlight differences. If we put these two people together, we would say that the louder one is Yang in relation to the quieter one. But—and there is always a but—if we put the meditating person next to a sleeping cat, the cat would be Yin in relation to the Yang meditator. If this cat wakes up and starts playing with papers while the person continues to meditate, the roles switch. This is the dance of Yin and Yang. Everything changes. Yin becomes Yang, Yang becomes Yin. Day becomes night, night becomes day. Everything is relative to something else.

In this medicine, health is reflected in the flowing, cooperative balance of Yin and Yang.

Qi

Qi ("chee") is another fundamental part of Chinese medicine. Qi is the energy of life. Qi enlivens everything. Without Qi, there is no life.

Qi is formless. Qi is the formless, unseen energy that animates every form. When Qi is abundant and flowing, the form that it animates reflects that energetic balance. When Qi is stagnant, excessive, or deficient, the form that it animates reflects this energetic imbalance.

Why do we need to understand the formless? Because manifestation arises from the formless Qi. In practicing our medicine, if we attend only to the form and not to the underlying Qi, we will never really "cure" the condition.

For example, a person diagnosed with high blood pressure, TMJ syndrome, and sciatica is prescribed a different medication for each condition. Additionally, they are working with a therapist to address their short, volcanic temper. Each of these four symptoms is a manifestation of an energetic disharmony that is easily identifiable within Chinese medicine. Rather than chasing four conditions with four medications, we could attend to the dynamics of the Wood Qi of this person. Working with specific meridians and points we can support the flow of Qi and the return to balance of Yin and Yang. With the restoring of harmony to the underlying energetic system, all four manifestations dissipate and the client has new resources to draw from as their life unfolds.

That an underlying Energy becomes manifested physically is one of the most challenging concepts for Western minds to grasp, understand, and know as a simple reality. To grasp this medicine, we must appreciate the movement from the formless to the formed as simply as we appreciate that apples fall from trees because of gravity.

Our challenge as ordinary humans who rely so heavily on our five senses to experience the world around us is to grasp the notions of Qi and Yin and Yang. If we are to practice Meridian Massage and understand Chinese medicine, we must set ourselves to the task of breaking through the limits of our senses and our intellect in order to know deeply in our cells that physical manifestation arises from an energetic basis. The state of that energetic basis will be reflected in the physical manifestation of our body.

Harmony

Harmonious energy gives rise to harmonious manifestations. Disharmonious energy gives rise to disorganized physical manifestations. Disorganized physical manifestations within a human body are referred to as symptoms and/or diseases. Chinese medicine seeks to harmonize the energetic foundation in order to alleviate disease/symptoms and support a healthy, vital, long life.

To be in harmony means to be in communication, in communion, in a constantly flowing mutually respectful and joyful relationship of yielding and instigating, rising and falling, giving and taking. Harmony among fifty players in an orchestra is reflected in the harmony of their music. Harmony between our organs, cells, and meridians is reflected in the harmonious expression of our joyful, flowing, healthy life.

Get Me Some Harmony!

The avenues of balancing and harmonizing energy, or Qi, from Classical Chinese medicine are many and include meditation, diet, lifestyle, physical exercise such as Qi Gong or Tai Chi, herbal medicine, massage, and acupuncture. Meridian Massage is one of many methods of harmonizing the Qi.

Each body, from the Chinese medical perspective, is a combination of Yin and Yang—of the Sky above us and the Earth below us—enlivened with Qi. Because Qi is the energetic source of our life and manifestation, it is the most logical place to attend to in order to sort out problems with the body. If we only address the physical body, the manifestation, we may never get to the root of the problem located in the Qi.

Is This a Little Confusing?

Of course it is. We are living a mystery. We don't have it all figured out at once. Our desire for answers sets us on a quest for knowledge and understanding. I trust that as long as I have this ball of confusion combined with curiosity and a desire for clarity, I must still be alive!

Here is a selection from the Tao Te Ching that helps settle my rattling mind:

> *Something mysteriously formed,*
> *Born before heaven and earth.*
> *In the silence and the void,*
> *Standing alone and unchanging,*
> *Ever present and in motion.*
> *Perhaps it is the mother of ten thousand things.*
> *I do not know its name.*
> *Call it Tao.*
> *For lack of a better word, I call it great.* [9]

The Tao Te Ching is a foundational book in Taoist philosophy. It was written thousands of years ago by the sage Lao Tzu (sometimes spelled as Lao Tsu, or Lao Zi). If you have a desire to be in contact with the origins of Classical Chinese medicine, I recommend keeping a copy with you for the years to come.

What Is the Nature of Qi?

Qi moves, flows, changes. The ever changing nature of Qi is reflected or referenced by the ever changing flow of Yin and Yang. We and our world are always changing. Have you noticed the change in season, in time, the temperature, your appetite, your thirst, your energy this week? Even if you haven't noticed, it has all changed.

We could say that Yin overtook Yang yesterday and night fell. We can say the Yang overtook Yin this morning as the Sun rose. Perhaps you can reflect that your Yang Qi was plentiful as you energetically sprang out of bed this morning. And later tonight, as you go with the flow of nature, when Yin once again takes over Yang at night, your Yin will expand as Yang decreases easily and you drop into a restful, quiet sleep.

Mind and Body

We think of minds as invisible, as not part of the body. But within this framework, mind and body are not separate—they are different densities of Qi. So, mental and emotional disharmonies also have their roots in stuck or disorganized Qi.

Mind is associated with the sky, vast, above, immaterial, Yang. Body is associated with the Earth, dense, formed, below, and Yin. Sky and Earth combine, Yin and Yang mingle, to create a human life. We are infused with these energies and so are in relation to them, even when we are not consciously aware of them. Qi energizes us, flows through us, takes on many different forms within us. Again and again, we move our thinking into a more "right brain," systemic, fluid, all-encompassing type of understanding.

Meridians

Qi flows through the body within meridians. These meridians cannot be seen, just as Qi itself cannot be seen. However, the meridians are located in anatomically precise lines throughout the body. Qi is stored, transformed, and released by Organs. Every meridian is rooted to an Organ.

Meridians are also referred to as channels.

It is by virtue of the twelve channels that human life
exists, that disease arises, that human beings can be treated
and illness cured. The twelve channels are where beginners
start and masters end. To beginners it seems easy; the
masters know how diffcult it is. [10]

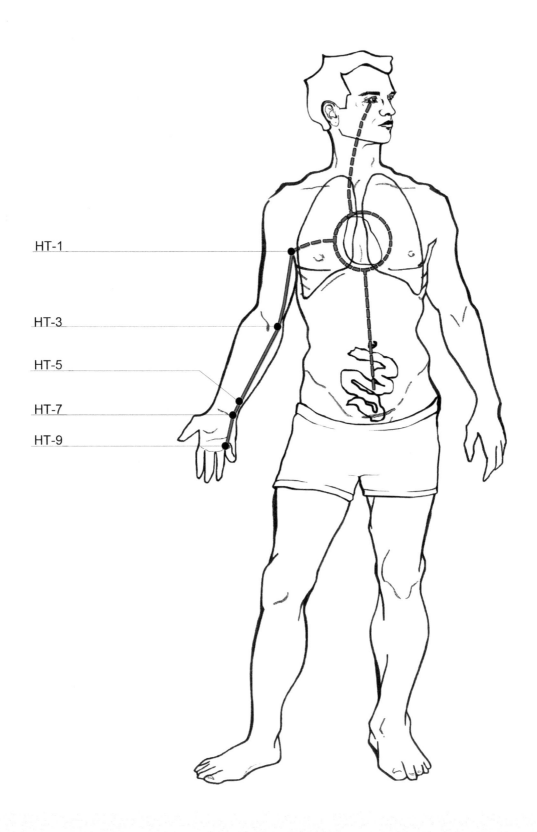

HT-1

HT-3

HT-5

HT-7

HT-9

HEART MERIDIAN

Think of a river. You might notice the water more obviously than the riverbed. The water flows within the riverbed. Which came first, the water or the river? This is an endless question. One answer is that the riverbed is where the water flows, and the water flows where the riverbed is.

Qi flows where the meridians are. The meridians are where the Qi flows.

Along the meridians are specific points. These points are located in reference to precise anatomical landmarks. The points are places along a meridian where the Qi is more readily accessed, where it can be "treated" or contacted in order to support its return to balanced flow. Just as we access a river at certain places along its path, we contact Qi at certain places along a meridian. These specific places where Qi can be accessed on a meridian are called "points" or "acupoints."

Originally the points were named. There are hundreds of regular points and many more "extra" points. Extra points are not located exactly on a meridian—many were identified after the original meridian map and points were settled on. In the West, points are referred to by numbers rather than names. In this book I reference the point names in Part 2, Chapter 1, Twelve Meridians. For ease, I use point numbers throughout the text.

As long as Qi is plentiful and flowing through all of the meridians, life is also balanced, harmonious, and joyous. Practitioners can utilize the flow of Qi in the meridians and at the points to directly support the rebalancing of Qi to resolve the root of physical ailments.

Qi flows both superficially, along the skin, and deep within every cell of the body. Meridians have internal pathways and external pathways. The external pathways are the pathways drawn on figures, and these are the pathways we work in massage.

Internal pathways connect to the Organ associated with the meridian. For example, the internal pathway of the Lung meridian connects with the physical lung organ. It also connects with the large intestine organ, which is the Yang pair of Lung meridian.

The internal pathways often solve the riddle of many effects that do not necessarily make sense if we base our thinking on only the external pathways of the meridians those effects are attributed to. Qi is delivered to every cell of the body along a web of meridian pathways.

Meridians are located on both sides and limbs of the body. It is traditional, as shown below, to depict the meridian (and points) on one side in order to allow the reader to visualize the pathway and its anatomical landmarks on the other side.

The main meridian pathways depicted on charts are like major highways on a map. If we look more closely at the road map, we will see smaller highways connecting to the interstates. Closer still we

In this diagram, the external pathway is the solid line, and the broken line signifies the internal pathway.

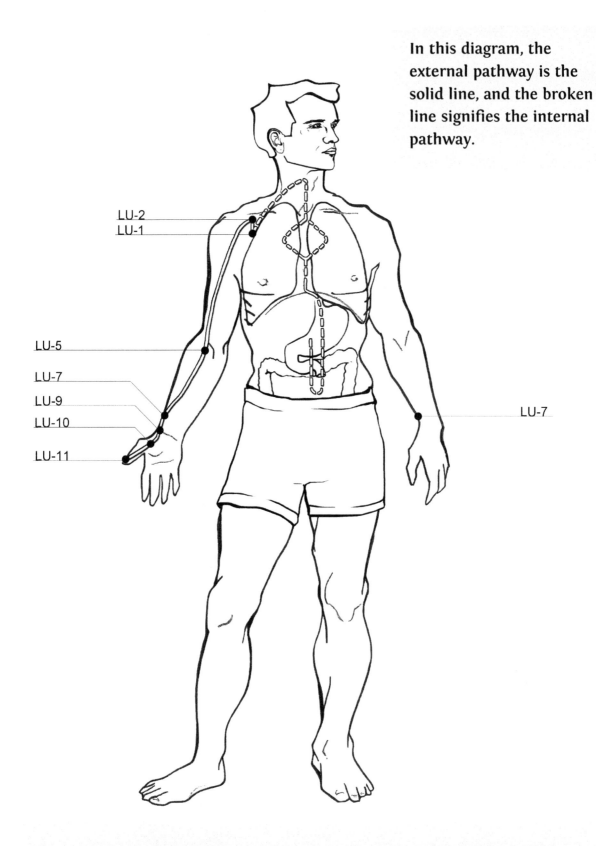

LU-2
LU-1

LU-5

LU-7
LU-9
LU-10

LU-11

LU-7

LUNG MERIDIAN SHOWING INTERNAL AND EXTERNAL PATHWAYS

see smaller yet active roads, and then we find the side roads. Not marked on maps are tiny driveways linking individual homes back to the interstate via a web of roads and highways.

Each meridian, or channel, is part of a web that includes all other meridians, and all their internal pathways. Meridians are "roads" of connection between organs, tissues, and other meridians, as well as pathways for the movement of Qi and Blood throughout the entire system.

Meridians Do Not Discriminate

Similar to roadways, meridians do not discriminate. Cops and robbers drive on the same roads. For this reason, meridians are pathways of "healthy" Qi as well as pathways for pathogens ("evil" or "pathogenic" Qi).

Wind is a common pathogen that can enter a meridian that is lacking in Qi. Once the Wind enters, it will travel along the pathway of the meridian. Clients will often trace the path of the meridian as they describe where their pain is. Following the path of their concern is one way we assess which meridian is affected.

This is similar to the Western notion of referred pain patterns.

Therapists use their knowledge of meridian pathways to assess the condition and treat it. By specifically focusing on the meridian, the therapist moves the Wind out of the meridian to make space for the return of healthy Qi. To accomplish this, the therapist will work with the whole meridian, with specific points on that meridian, and with points on other meridians associated with the issue.

For example, Wind in the Gallbladder meridian may arise as a pattern of pain from the hip and down the outside of the same leg. In Western medicine this condition may be termed "sciatica." Chinese medicine may classify it as Wind blocking the Gallbladder meridian. To resolve this pain we would massage specific points on the Gallbladder to encourage the release of Wind out of the meridian and the return of flowing Qi. When the Wind is released and the Qi is once again flowing, the "sciatic" pain will disappear.

Meridian Massage

What is Meridian Massage actually doing? When you realize that a meridian is not really a "thing" but a pathway for energy, it is kind of funny to consider massaging one. Thousands of years ago meridians were somehow discovered and mapped out. The course of time has proven the reality of meridians and Qi, and the wisdom of working with them.

Meridians and points can be treated in many different ways. Chinese medicine uses needles, massage, herbs, exercise, moxibustion (heat), cupping, meditation, and diet and lifestyle adjustments to affect the Qi in the meridians.

Meridian Massage is not a formal method of Chinese medicine. It is a modern hands-on approach to working with Qi. When we "massage" meridians, we are focusing on the energy, the Qi of our client. The ultimate intention of Meridian Massage is to support abundant, free-flowing, harmonized Qi. Abundant, free-flowing, and harmonized Qi is the energetic basis of physical, mental, and emotional health and well-being.

Using the meridians as pathways, we support our clients' increased awareness of their inner worlds and Qi. It is within this inner world that each of us "meets ourself." These meetings, or meeting points, provide the possibility for integrating Yin and Yang, right brain and left brain, conscious and unconscious, masculine and feminine, body and mind, form and formless. As our energies are literally unblocked and reconnected with each other, our Qi flows, the Organs are nourished and function optimally. We enjoy vitality, energy strength, and flexibility in our body-mind-emotions-spirit.

Body Structure, Organ Systems, and Meridians

An Organ is considered to be a complete system that includes the physical organ, its associated meridian, tissue, Element, body area, sense organ, taste, season, color, sound, two-hour time period within the twenty-four hours of a day, and emotion. Because this idea of an organ is so vastly different than that of Western science, when referring to organs in Chinese medicine, the terms are capitalized. For example, when referring to the kidney organ system, Chinese medicine would write "Kidney" rather than "kidney."

Chinese anatomy includes all of the muscles, bones, nerves, blood vessels, etc. At the center of Chinese anatomy are the meridians. Meridians are part of the web of Organ systems. Organ systems are associated with a particular type of Qi and with each Organ. There is no separation between the physical organ and its Qi.

Think of a friend of yours. When you think of this person, you actually consider many things about them—their physical body, whom they might be in a relationship with, their job, their general outlook on life, the sound of their voice, color of their skin, their family, where they live—all of these things are combined together in your sense of this person. This way of thinking is systemic. You are able to hold many types of information about a single person all at once—it just makes sense.

We must develop this kind of sense of Organ systems in order to understand the body as viewed by Chinese medicine. In this way, when you think of Kidney, you will immediately consider the kidney organs, bones, low back area, the Kidney and Bladder meridians, water, winter, ears, fear, salty, groaning, blue, black, all at the same time—simple!

Later we will explore each Organ system in detail. For now, the goal is to open your mind to the notion of Qi, Energy, as being the basis from which the body manifests. The brilliance of this system of medicine is how it fully incorporates Qi into its understanding of health, illness, and recovery.

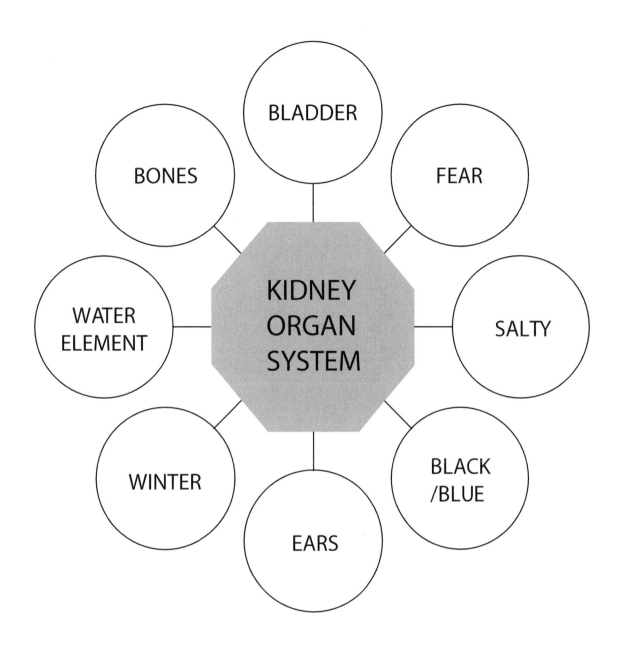

KIDNEY ORGAN SYSTEM

By observing Nature, we are able to attune ourselves to the same body of knowledge that the ancients pondered in order to synthesize this medicine. We benefit directly from their dedication and skill as we enter into our own study of Meridian Massage. We honor the knowledge that has been passed down and preserved by so many compassionate practitioners as we persevere in our own study of this brilliant health system and well-being today.

2: Four Building Blocks

1. Shen
2. Essence
3. Qi
4. Blood

All cultures ponder the same human organism. Yet we all come up with different ideas of what we are, why we are here, how our body is structured, and how it functions. Within the framework of Chinese medicine, Shen, Essence, Qi, and Blood can be thought of as four foundational aspects or "building blocks" of a human being.

In this worldview, Nature holds the Mystery of where we come from, what we are made of, and our purpose as individuals and as a species. It includes plants, animals, and bugs as well as space, time, the universe, gravity, and more. It is seen in the various manifestations of life. It is unseen as the originator of all life.

From this Nature, all things arise and one day return. Out of the unseen aspect of Nature spring Yin and Yang. From that essential duality of interdependent forces comes everything, including humans. Humans are a precious combination of Yin and Yang, endowed with Shen, Essence, Qi, and Blood.

Shen

Shen is often translated as "Spirit." It is immaterial and eternal. Shen is consciousness in our broadest sense of the term. It is the highest "ideal" of ourselves. When we are asked to rise to an occasion and we see ourselves acting in ways that are virtuous beyond our everyday activity, we are sensing our Shen and acting from it.

We get a glimpse of how we could really be, of what we aspire in our heart of hearts to become. Shen is always a part of us, always present even though we may not be in conscious contact with this aspect of ourselves. Shen is that in us which is closest to the unseen Mystery of Nature. It is our own little "spark of star dust," our scaled-down expression of the vast unseen Mystery of Nature.

Shen is Yang (energetic, immaterial) in relationship to Essence, which is Yin (material, dense). Shen and Essence are an essential Yin-Yang pair within the human.

Essence

At conception we get our Essence. In the West, we say that at conception we get our DNA - half from the egg, half from the sperm.

Essence is the most "material" or densest form of the unseen Mystery of Nature that we have. It is the "drop" of something from nothing that is the basis of our creation. From the Essence we build our Blood and Qi. From the Blood and Qi, we build our physical form. This is why Essence is so precious: It is the basis of our physical life.

It is challenging to sense Essence as material. It is not material in the way that a counter top is. It is material in relationship to Shen.

What is DNA? A molecule. What is a molecule? How do we become physical in the Western view? DNA drives every cellular program. How did the donut and coffee we ate for breakfast become new muscle fiber after our workout? Digestion breaks down and sends the nutrient to the cell. DNA directs the formation of proteins from amino acids. Recall DNA and RNA and building the strands of protein. Sometimes the repetition of this story makes it seem that DNA is somehow solid and "real." Yet DNA is a molecule—not so solid after all.

Essence is denser than Spirit—yet not a solid material "thing."

These are different stories for the same phenomenon.

We have a set amount of Essence from conception. When that Essence runs out, so does our physical life. When the physical life ends, the Shen departs.

The quality of Essence is reflected in our general constitution. You assess this when you evaluate an individual as lively, dull, smart, healthy, tired, weak, strong, etc.

Qi

There is a famous axiom: "Qi is the Commander of Blood, and Blood is the Mother of Qi."
Qi is Yang in relationship to Yin Blood. Qi is our energy that flows through the meridians and Organs.

Qi is denser than Shen on a continuum from immaterial to material. Qi is "coarser" and more immediately felt than Shen.

Qi relies on Blood for a place to "live." I imagine Blood as the "body of Qi." Without Blood, Qi has no place to land, no substance to keep it firmly held, no form. Qi moves the Blood through the vessels and meridians. Qi is spoken of as the force of the Blood–what could that mean? Think of the power of the heart contraction to move the blood. What is the "power?" It is Qi.

Qi enlivens us, keeps us warm, stimulates all functions in the body.

Blood

Consider again the famous axiom: "Qi is the Commander of Blood, and Blood is the Mother of Qi."

This is an important concept to understand. Blood is material, Yin, nourishing, and essential to life. Qi is energetic, Yang, moving, and essential to life. Thinking along the continuum of material to immaterial, we can conceive of Blood as the material aspect of Qi, or Qi as the immaterial aspect of Blood.

Blood is liquid, lubricating, moist. These Yin qualities of Blood ensure the flexibility and ease of movement of our bones, muscles, tendons, and ligaments. The interdependency of these two is the central message of the axiom.

Notice that Blood is capitalized here to signify that in this context Blood includes what we know as blood and more–just like with Organ and organ. Blood includes the nurturing, lubricating, energetic quality of the physical manifestation.

The Blood provides the material, the vessel, for the Qi to "swim" in. Without Blood, Qi has no place to reside and will drift away. Feel the similarity here to the Spirit (Yang) needing the Body (Yin) to reside in.

The Blood will not stay in the vessels, nor can it move, without the presence of Qi. Qi is the force that moves Blood. Think of the Heart pumping the blood, the Qi is the "pump" of the Blood. Without Qi and Blood there is no life.

Although there is constant reference to Qi, we must always keep in mind the essential substance of Blood.

Blood is created from Essence combined with Qi. The Spleen is an essential player in the quality and quantity of Blood as it must absorb Qi and nutrients from the food we eat. The Heart governs the Blood and the blood vessels. The Liver stores the Blood at night. The Blood is Yin compared to Qi.

At night, the Blood nourishes us and provides the resting place for Qi and the Mind. If the Blood is not plentiful, our sleep is restless, our Mind has no place to rest.

Women naturally have more Blood than men, who naturally have more Qi than women. This reflects the Yin nature of women and Yang nature of men. It does not say that women have no Qi or that men have no Blood, it speaks to relative balance. Indeed, balance for everyone includes the individual's balance of Yin and Yang, masculine and feminine, Blood and Qi, etc.

These four are one.

Although treated as separate "things," Shen, Essence, Qi, and Blood are all manifestations of the same "thing." This singular "thing" is a thread of the Mysterious Source of Nature from which everything arises.

Shen	Qi	Blood	Essence

From immaterial to material

These four aspects are also Yang and Yin pairs as shown below

YANG	YIN
Shen	Essence
Qi	Blood

3: The Five Elements or Transformations

Conceptually it is helpful to think of the Five Elements as five seasons. Five in this context is confusing as we recognize four seasons. It is said that there are "four seasons and Five Elements" (Yellow Emperor's Classic of Medicine). By adding "Late Summer"—that time between summer and fall that can be warm and humid—we get five seasons and Five Elements.

Notice that each season has certain characteristics that we can count on. We know it's going to be cold in the winter and warm in the summer. Things sprout in spring and leaves drop in the fall. The seasons are identifiable even though we are constantly cycling through them. This is how to understand the Five Elements.

Each Element is recognizable, but not a stagnant "thing" unto itself. Because of the cycling through the Elements by season, these are often referred to as "transformations." Humans, as the microcosmic reflection of a macrocosmic Universe have these same Five Elements within us.

Every Organ system is associated with a particular Element, as are tastes, colors, seasons, emotions, and more. The table to the right outlines key associations to know about each Element.

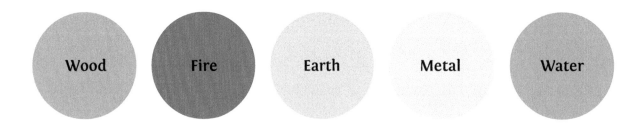

Element	Wood	Fire	Earth	Metal	Water
Season	Spring	Summer	Late Summer	Fall	Winter
Yang Organ	Gallbladder	Small Intestine San Jiao	Stomach	Large Intestine	Bladder
Yin Organ	Liver	Heart Pericardium	Spleen	Lung	Kidney
Emotion	Anger / Kindness	Hyper Extroversion / Joy	Worry / Satisfaction	Grief / Courage	Fear / Creativity
Sense Organ	Eyes	Tongue	Mouth / Lips	Nose	Ears
Tissue	Tendons	Blood	Muscles	Skin	Bone
Weather	Wind	Heat	Humid / Damp	Dry	Cold
Action	Growing	Showing / Sharing	Manifesting	Letting Go	Incubating
Cycle of a plant	Sprout	Flower	Fruit	Seeds Drop	Store, Incubate seed, End and beginning of the cycle

Getting to the Five Elements

Things manifest from an energetic Source or Mystery of Nature that is unseen, vast, and living. This Source is undifferentiated. In order for things to appear, first something "triggers" this Source to differentiate out Yin and Yang. From Yin and Yang, all things further differentiate into the Five Elements. From the Five Elements, manifestations arise in keeping with a variety of cycles.

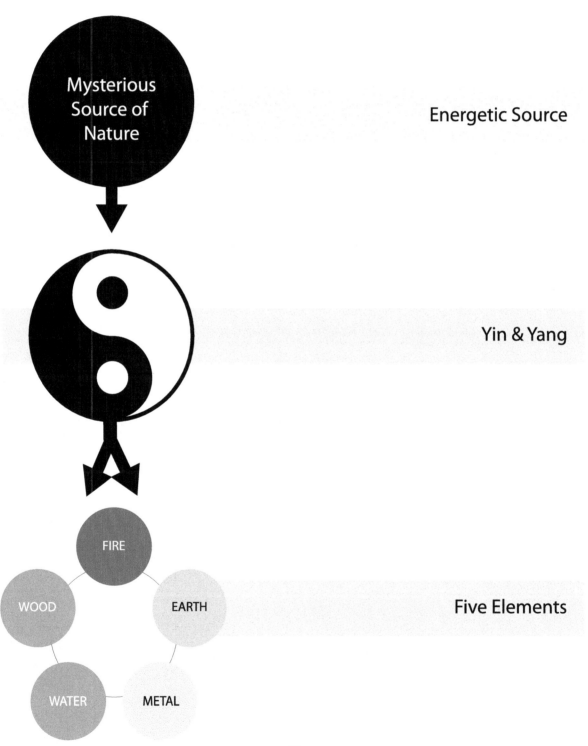

Energetic Source

Yin & Yang

Five Elements

Yin and Yang are the foundational energies from which everything else arises. The figure below shows the movement of Yin and Yang.

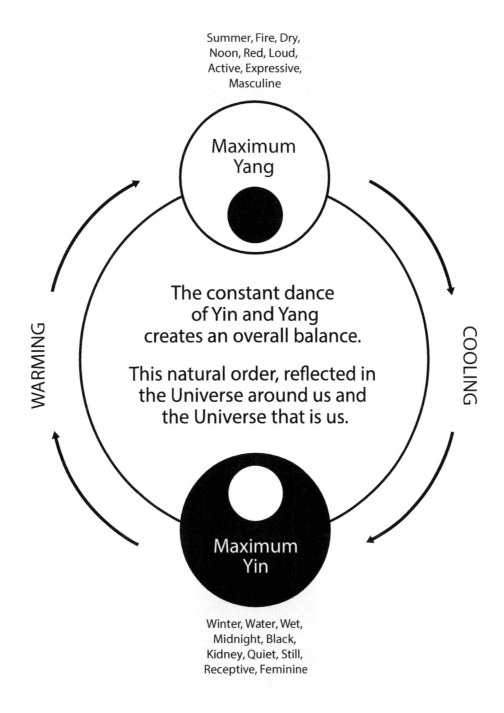

Summer, Fire, Dry,
Noon, Red, Loud,
Active, Expressive,
Masculine

Maximum
Yang

WARMING

COOLING

The constant dance
of Yin and Yang
creates an overall balance.

This natural order, reflected in
the Universe around us and
the Universe that is us.

Maximum
Yin

Winter, Water, Wet,
Midnight, Black,
Kidney, Quiet, Still,
Receptive, Feminine

At the extreme (maximum), Yang turns into Yin, and Yin will transform into Yang. Night becomes day, day becomes night. Winter becomes Summer, Summer becomes Winter.

A further division of Yin and Yang shows us four seasons and Yin-Yang balance within them (Summer and Winter, Spring and Fall):

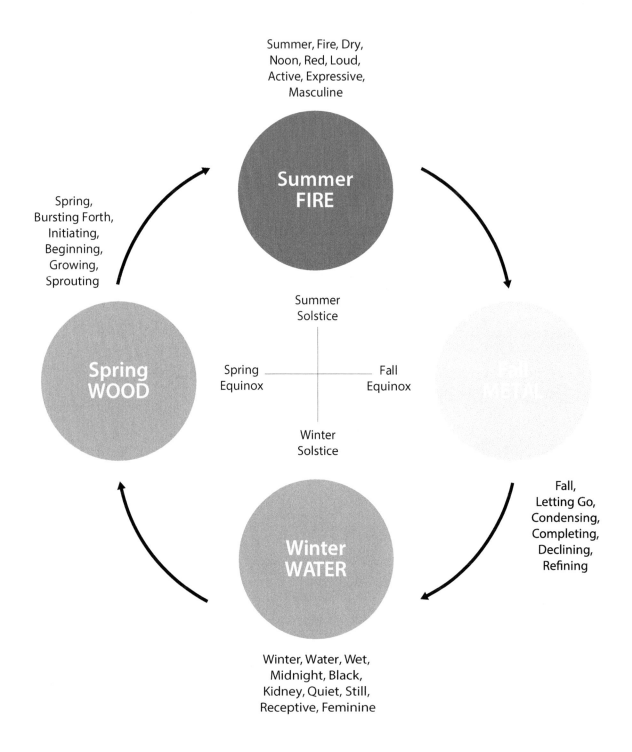

THE CYCLE OF FOUR SEASONS

Each season corresponds to an Element. We come to Five Seasons or the Five Elements by adding in Late Summer:

Winter—Water
Spring—Wood
Summer—Fire
Late Summer—Earth
Fall—Metal

The figure below shows the "Creation cycle," which flows in the same order as the cycle of the Seasons:

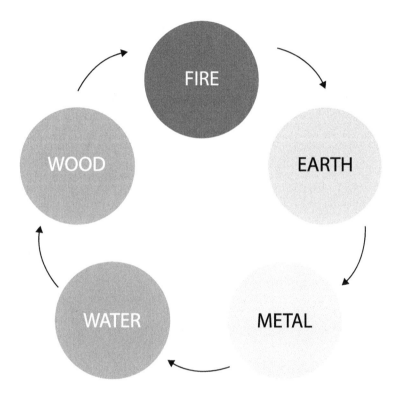

GENERATING CYCLE, ALSO KNOWN AS CREATION CYCLE

The Creation cycle shows us how each Element nurtures the next Element. In this cycle, the Elements are encouraged to grow and expand. The Creation cycle is also referred to as the "Mother-Child" cycle. For example, Wood is the Mother of Fire as Wood is the fuel of Fire, thus helping Fire burn and grow. Using the seasons to help our understanding, winter becomes spring could be imagined as winter is the Mother of spring, or winter creates spring. And spring creates summer, summer creates late summer, and so forth.

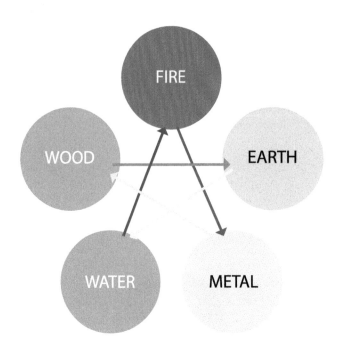

THE CONSOLIDATION CYCLE, ALSO KNOWN AS THE CONTROL CYCLE

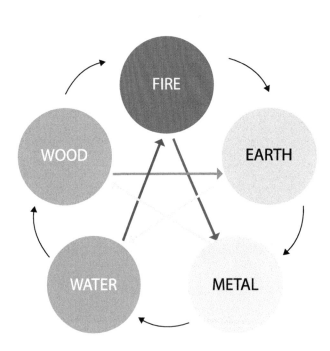

CYCLE OF THE FIVE TRANSFORMATIONS: GENERATING AND CONSOLIDATION

Opposite in nature from the Creation cycle, the Consolidation cycle (left, top) limits the growth or expansion of the Elements. This cycle is sometimes referred to the Grandparents cycle.

Putting these two cycles together produces the "Creation and Consolidation cycle" (left, bottom).

Here we see how balance is maintained through the relationships of the Five Elements. Expansion and growth are Yang attributes compared to Yin reduction and consolidation. When Yin and Yang are harmonized, moving, and balancing each other, all of the Five Elements remain harmonious as well.

It is also easy to see that if just one Element grows too large or too small, the balance of the whole system is thrown off. From this point of view, there is no difference between the energetics of the Elements and the energetics of the Organs, the meridians, and the associations with the Organ.

How can we support the balance of these Five Elements? By working with the Qi in the meridians and Organs.

The physical body is a manifestation of energy. Organ systems are "crossroads" between the physical body and the energy that manifests, animates, sustains, and transforms the body. Much more than simply physical "things," Organs in Chinese medicine are webs of energetic and physical phenomena. Again, to emphasize the difference between the physical-body organ and these energy systems, we capitalize the word "Organ" when referring to an Organ system from the Chinese perspective.

Wood Element

SEASON: Spring
YIN ORGAN: Liver
YANG ORGAN: Gallbladder
SENSE ORGAN: Eyes
TISSUE: Ligaments and tendons
COLOR: Green
WEATHER: Wind

Wood Element in Nature

Spring marks the birth of a new cycle of growth. Out of the stillness of winter, movement returns. The Wood Element is all about growth and expansion as it is the beginning of the warming-up cycle, the movement from Yin to Yang. Having passed through the coldest time of the year, things begin to warm up as the light of the Sun returns, the days grow longer, plants begin to shoot up through the soil, animals give birth to babies.

Plants and trees are literal manifestations of the Wood Element.

Wood Element in Humans

Our birth and youth mark the "spring" of our lifetime. Children bursting forth with fresh, wild, abundant energy, full of curiosity and ready for action. Wood Energy is active, outward, expansive, growing.

The eyes are the sense organ of the Wood Element. Visionaries see things before they even begin. They prompt us and inspire us to new action, to try new things. Wood Energy guides the way, insisting that the "impossible" is indeed possible.

Trees gently swaying in the wind rely on the strength of their trunk and roots to hold them up. In humans, we rely on our tendons and ligaments to hold our skeleton upright.

A soft breeze is enjoyable. Too much wind can harm, but no wind feels stuffy and heavy. Wind penetrates every open crack in a home. Wind can invade the meridian system if there is not enough Qi filling the meridians. Wind is often the first climatic factor to invade the meridians. Wind easily creates an opening for other external pathogens. Wind that invades from the outside is termed "External Wind."

Internal Wind is generated within the Liver Organ system when it is overwhelmed. Excess internal Wind manifests as twitching and fidgeting, just like the wind through the leaves of a tree. Larger excesses of Wind are like a tornado or hurricane within the body, manifesting as heart attacks or strokes. Complete lack of Wind, paralysis, is the extreme outcome of excess Wind injuring the brain in a stroke.

We all need some Wind. A gentle breeze to keep the air flowing in a room and the Qi flowing through the meridians. This is why it is said that the Liver is responsible to ensure the smooth flow of Qi through the meridians.

Wood Element within the Cycle of the Five Elements

Generating Cycle
Wood nourishes Fire.
Wood is the fuel for Fire. In order for Fire to exist, it must have Wood to burn.

Wood is nourished by the Water Element.
Just as for plants drawing water into their roots, our Wood Energy is nourished by our Water Element. Without enough Water, the Wood Element will suffer. If our Kidneys (Yin Organ of the Water Element) are exhausted, they will not be able to support the Liver. The Liver grows the seeds of creativity held in the Kidneys. If there is nothing in the Kidneys, there is nothing to grow.

Consolidation Cycle
The Wood Element consolidates the Earth Element.
Just as the roots of trees and plants hold a hillside in place, our tendons anchor the muscles (tissue of the Earth Element) to the bones.

The weather condition of the Earth Element is dampness and humidity. Wind dissipates humidity or "controls" the excess dampness of Earth.

Metal Consolidates Wood.
Just as Wood loves to expand, Metal loves to cut back, to trim. We use axes and saws made out of metal to cut down trees and mow the lawn. The growth of Wood is held in check by Metal. Imagine our world if every person, plant, and animal only grew more and more, never stopping! The relief of resting after work, the clear feeling after cleaning out a cluttered closet is the balance that Metal brings to Wood.

Fire Element

SEASON: Summer
YIN ORGAN: Heart
YANG ORGAN: Small Intestine
SENSE ORGAN: Tongue
TISSUE: Blood
COLOR: Red
WEATHER: Hot

Fire is the only Element with four Organs (and therefore four meridians). Fire is subdivided into Cardinal Fire and Supplemental Fire.

• Cardinal Fire: Heart (Yin) and Small Intestine (Yang)
• Supplemental Fire: Pericardium (Yin) and San Jiao (Yang)

Comparing Cardinal Fire and Supplemental Fire:
The attributes of passion, expansion, and spreading warmth and light are more attributed to Cardinal Fire. The Heart Organ is said to be the Emperor, who oversees all other Organs. Think of the ultra-importance of an Emperor of a vast country—this is the energy of Cardinal Fire and the Heart Organ.

The attribute of communication is more attributed to Supplemental Fire. The sense organ of the Fire Element is the tongue, which relates to speaking and communicating. We also communicate with ourselves. Physiologically, a great deal of communication is carried out by our hormones. Hormones and internal communication are attributed to the Pericardium and San Jiao.

Fire Element in Nature

The Sun represents the largest Fire in Nature. The Sun lights the entire sky and Earth, bringing warmth, renewal, and light. Fire itself offers warmth and light. Summer is the season of warmth, being outdoors, visiting with others.

In summer, the flowers are in full bloom, baby animals are transitioning out of the nest, vegetables are plump and ripening.

Fire Element in Humans

Fire captures our attention. Notice how people are almost mesmerized by a campfire or a burning candle. When the fire is gone, so is our interest—how often do you gaze dreamlike at an unlit candle?

Imagine people as candles. The height of the flame can be observed in their general physical and emotional warmth, the amount and volume that they speak, their overall "glow," ability to connect and communicate with new people. The bigger the flame, the more charisma and expression of joy. The lower the flame, the quieter and more inward and self-contained.

The Element that brings up our hopes, dreams, passion, warm feelings and sense of community is Fire.

Fire literally keeps us warm. The amount of physical warmth (or lack of warmth) a person experiences reflects the state of their Fire Element. Fire is literally red. The red–pink–bright glow of happiness is Fire.

Fire Element within the Cycle of the Five Elements

Generating Cycle
Fire nourishes Earth. It is a common practice to burn land in order to revive it. Soon after a field or forest is burned, fresh new growth springs up. Fire also warms and brightens our Earth Element in the same way that the Sun warms the Earth.

Fire is nourished by Wood.
Wood is the fuel of Fire.

Consolidation Cycle

Fire consolidates Metal.
Fire can melt Metal so it can be forged into many useful tools. The warmth and love of Fire soothes the cold, dense, rigid boundary that Metal can form, blocking us off from our relations and our community. When another person's presence and love melts our boundaries and we feel the relief of expressing our emotions and the ability to again connect with others, we are experiencing the balancing effect of Fire melting Metal.

Fire is consolidated by Water.
Fire can burn fast and wide. Water is the Element that contains Fire, dampens it, keeps it in check. People everywhere know to throw water on fire to reduce its size.

Too much Fire can burn up all of the fuel. When a roaring Fire has nothing left to burn, it "goes out," meaning it dies.

Fire is the ultimate Yang of the body, Water is the ultimate Yin of the body. These two forces are in a constant dance of dependence with one another. Fire and Water must balance each other to offer the essential harmony upon which the entire organism depends.

Even though we are discussing the Five Element Cycle, always keep in mind that behind it, or prior to the Five Elements are the two essentials: Yin and Yang, Water and Fire.

Earth Element

SEASON: Late Summer and the transitions between all seasons
YIN ORGAN: Spleen (and Pancreas)
YANG ORGAN: Stomach
SENSE ORGAN: Lips
TISSUE: Muscles
COLOR: Yellow
WEATHER: Damp and Humid

Earth Element in Nature

Earth is our planet, our home, the fertile ground beneath us. The Earth gives all life a place to live. It provides a place to be and the soils from which all plants grow. All life is dependent upon the Earth for a place to live and for ongoing nourishment to live.

The Earth nourishes all life and recycles or composts all material that is left after life. Always under us, supporting us, nourishing us, providing a home for all that we know as our place or home.

Earth Element in Humans

The Me, as an Infinite Spirit, needs a place to "be" in the material world in order to express as an individual. Our Body is our home, our place of physical manifestation. The physical body provides a home to the Spirit just as the Earth provides a home to all life forms.

Muscles are the tissue of the Earth Element, providing the bulk of our home. Just as the Earth provides nourishment as well as recycling and composting, our digestive system receives food, breaks it down, churns it, absorbs it, and "feeds" this material to our cells. The Stomach is said to "rot and ripen" the food. The Spleen absorbs the Qi from the processed food.

We must be able nourish ourselves by means of digestion to keep our physical body alive, providing a home to the Spirit. Our abilities to receive nourishment and give nourishment are fundamental Earth Element qualities.

Mothers provide, in their wombs, the first home to babies. Mothers first must have enough food to provide the nutrients required for growth and development from conception to birth. Mothering, nurturing, providing for others, sharing, generosity are Earth Element topics.

Presence is an Earth quality. Being present, available, and responsive to our life mirrors the unending presence of the Earth beneath us, always supporting us and giving us a place to live.

Earth Element within the Cycle of the Five Elements

Generating Cycle

Earth nourishes Metal.
Earth is the container of Metal. Different types of metal ore are often located deep inside the earth.

Earth is nourished by Fire.
Ash is a source of nourishment for soil. Burning fields is an age-old practice to promote new growth and to build up the soil.

Consolidation Cycle

Earth consolidates Water.
Ponds are limited or held by the earth. We can dam up a river using earth. Without a container, water spreads and oozes unchecked. Earth provides a container for Water.

Earth is consolidated by Wood.
The roots of plants and trees hold the earth, keeping it from sliding away in floods or blowing away in droughts.

Metal Element

SEASON: Fall
YIN ORGAN: Lungs
YANG ORGAN: Large Intestine
SENSE ORGAN: Nose
TISSUE: Skin
COLOR: White
WEATHER: Dry

Metal Element in Nature

Minerals and metals such as calcium, copper, iron, etc., are found throughout Nature in many different forms. From massive copper mines to the invisible minerals of our body, Metal is there quietly playing an essential role to life.

Metal is hard, quiet, contained, steady, and usually found inside other material. Fall is the season of Metal, it is the beginning of Yin, of going inward, retreating, the letting-go of leaves, descending inward in preparation for Winter. In the Fall, the nests are empty, the air is dry and cool, plant material that gave so much during the summer is disintegrating back into the ground, seeds are dropping, the days are noticeably shorter as Yin begins to dominate the twenty-four-hour cycle.

All of the creation, expansion, enjoyment, and satisfaction of the previous seasons has come to an end. It is a time of reflection in preparation for the next cycle.

Metal Element in Humans

Metal gives us boundary in the form of our skin. It also gives us the ability to feel ourselves via our skin. Self-reflection and bringing the attention inward are the gifts of awareness to our breath. Meditation and contemplation are practices of the Metal Element.

The Lungs (Yin Organ of the Metal Element) breathe in essential oxygen and Qi needed for every cell.

Fall is a time of letting-go, becoming quiet, still, and inwardized in contrast to the expansive qualities of Spring (Wood Element). The Large Intestine is the Yang Organ of the Metal Element. Our ability to let go of what is not essential is reflected in the process of elimination via bowel movements.

Our ability to be in touch with ourselves, to reflect, and to contemplate our past in order gain wisdom is similar to saving the precious seeds from the withering plants of Fall for next year.

Metal Element within the Cycle of the Five Elements

Generating Cycle

Metal nourishes Water.
Minerals provide passageways for water deep in the earth.

Metal is nourished by Earth.
The earth holds minerals deep inside. Think of diamonds forming within the earth.

Consolidation Cycle

Metal consolidates Wood.
Metal cuts Wood, as in axes, lawnmowers, or pruning shears. Metal limits the growth of Wood.

Metal is consolidated by Fire.
Fire melts Metal, making it possible to change its form and function.

Water Element

SEASON: Winter
YIN ORGAN: Kidneys
YANG ORGAN: Bladder
SENSE ORGAN: Ears
TISSUE: Bones
COLOR: Blue and Black
WEATHER: Cold

Water Element in Nature

Water flows in all directions to the lowest level. Water is vast as the ocean and tiny as a raindrop. Water has no boundaries except those imposed upon it by something such as a glass, a dam, stones, the earthen shore. Water has many forms from ice to fluid to steam. Although it flows to low places, water also rises up to the sky when heated by the Sun.

Water is Yin in relation to the Yang of Fire. Water and Fire balance each other.

In Taoism, the philosophical basis of Classical Chinese Medicine, Water is held in high regard. Water is often used as a metaphor for the Tao. The following lines are from verse 8 of the Tao Te Ching:

> *The highest good is like water.*
> *Water gives life to the ten thousand things and does not strive.*
> *It flows in places men reject and so is like the Tao.*[11]

Winter, the coldest, darkest time of the year, is the season of the Water Element. Although above ground it seems as if nothing is happening, below the ground seeds are incubating.

This is a time of stillness, incubation, the creative time of inspiration prior to the emergence of creative impulse.

Water Element in Humans

The Kidneys are the Yin Organs of the Water Element. Our Life Force, or Essence, is held in the Kidneys. The Kidneys govern reproduction. Male and female reproductive organs are governed by the Kidneys. Similar to the seeds protected and incubated beneath the ground in winter, sperm and egg are the seeds of human creation. As we realize the potential of creation of sperm and egg, we get a glimpse into the potential creativity of the Water Element.

Our Essence is our literal connection to our ancestors. We receive DNA, Essence, at the moment of conception. This Essence has been passed down through hundreds of generations.

An ocean could be thought of as a mass of individual water drops merged into a massive single unit called "the ocean." In this context, the water is undifferentiated, merged, unified, "one." Staying with this metaphor, our individual expression of this lifetime is similar to a drop of water that has separated from the ocean. For a time, the drop is separated from the one, now individualized, yet destined always to return back to the ocean.

An individual human is a seemingly independent expression of a unified whole of undifferentiated energy or potential. This undifferentiated potential is referred to as the Tao in Taoism. From this perspective, our life is much more than we can fathom with our five senses, and much more than this particular lifetime.

You might notice that we are drifting into a topic that seems endless, mysterious, hard to explain. This is the depth and darkness of Water, of Yin. Compared to the differentiated, bright daytime expression of Yang, Yin is murky, internal, mysterious, wordless.

The Water Element "marks" both death and life. The Elements are transitions, they are not static moments. From the perspective of Taoism, upon which this medicine is based, death marks the letting-go of the body, but the Spirit continues.

Water Element within the Cycle of the Five Elements

Generating Cycle

Water generates Wood.
Plants and trees rely on water to grow. Notice what you do when you see your house plant wilting in the heat—you give it some water. Wood is the avenue for Water to move up toward the sky. The creative force of Water manifests upwardly and outwardly in the Wood Element.

Water is nourished by Metal.
Metal gives minerals to Water. Think of the difference between fresh spring water or mineral water compared to "city water."

Consolidation Cycle

Water consolidates Fire.

Water contains or even puts out Fire. Water is Yin in relation to the Yang of Fire. Water and Fire are the essential Yin-Yang axis within the human energetic matrix.

Water is consolidated by Earth.
Earth gives boundaries to Water.

It's all about balance

Expanding and contracting, warming and cooling, drying and wetting, growing and declining, doing and being—all of these describe polarities. There is no judgement in them, they are only descriptors. Within these descriptions there is nothing inherently better in one aspect of the polarity than the other.

The central concept is to be able to discern each quality of a pair and move toward a balance of both. Excess or deficiency of either is out of balance and will throw off the harmony of the entire system. Balance is not a rigid state of maintaining a perfect center point of any of these pairs—it is the ability to be aware and responsive to the changes. Seasons change, demanding changes from us, for instance wearing lighter clothes in the summer and heavier in the winter.

We change as our lives progress. How we respond to the changing seasons of Nature changes as our age changes. Balance in this sense means being able to make an appropriate "balancing" responses.

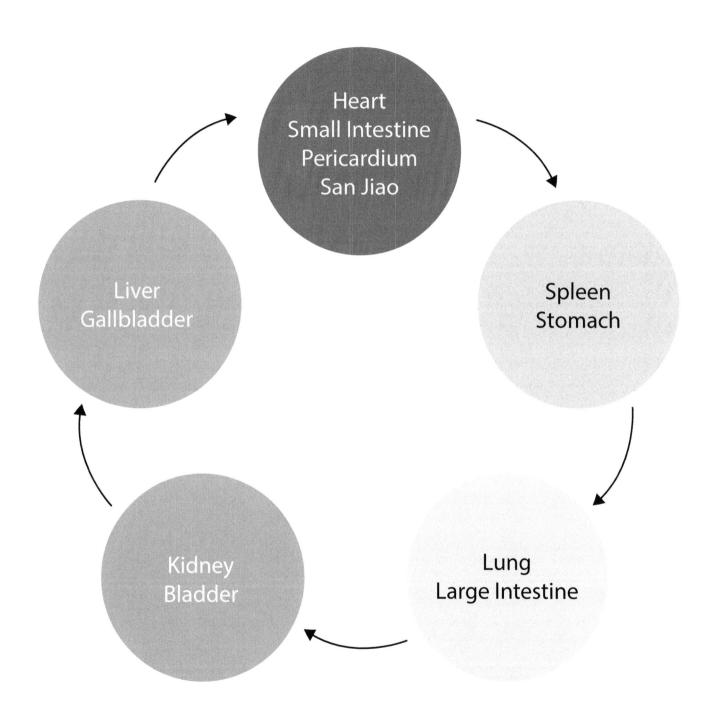

4: Organ Systems

Yin and Yang

Everything in Chinese medicine, including the Organs, is classified within the Yin and Yang perspective. Yin Organs hold and transform Qi. Yin Organs ultimately provide the nourishment for every aspect of the body.

Yang Organs transport Qi throughout the network of Organs. They also transport physical substances, such as food and water, through the physical body. The bladder and gastrointestinal tract are made up of Yang Organs. These Organs collectively receive food and water transporting this material through the system and excreting what is not used.

Yin and Yang Organs are paired. These pairs may seem strange at first glance, but with continued study one comes to appreciate the wisdom of these categorizations.

Each Organ pair is further categorized within the framework of the Five Elements of Fire, Earth, Metal, Water, and Wood. The discussion of Organs is incomplete without reference to the Elements, and the discussion of the Elements is incomplete without reference to the Organs. Studying the Organs and the Elements in their many relationships requires repetition, perseverance, curiosity, and patience.

You will need to refer to the preceding chapter on the Elements to fully understand the Organ systems and vice versa. We have to start somewhere, so let's begin with the Organs.

Yin and Yang Organ Pairs of Classical Chinese Medicine

Organs are systems within which the physical organ itself plays a role not necessarily larger than any of the other associated parts. In the West, for example, we are used to thinking only of the physical manifestation of a muscular pump when we hear reference to the anatomical heart. But within the energetic framework of Chinese medicine the term "Heart" refers to a system. Each Organ system includes, at a minimum: an organ, a season, an Element, an emotion, a taste, a color, a tissue, a sense organ, a Yang partner Organ, and a meridian.

YIN	YANG
Liver	Gallbladder
Heart	Small Intestine
Pericardium	San Jiao
Spleen	Stomach
Lung	Large Intestine
Kidney	Bladder

The associations with each Organ system are the basis of understanding human physiology from the Chinese perspective. In order to evaluate and treat imbalances of Qi, we must understand the flow and manifestation of Qi throughout the Organ systems. Qi, energy, arises as a set of manifestations (tissue, color, sense organ, taste, etc.) gathered around the central physical manifestation of an Organ.

Because the Yin Organs are central to acquiring, transforming, and maintaining the Qi, they hold a more significant stature than the Yang Organs. For this reason, when speaking about Organ systems, the Yin Organ is the main reference rather than the Yang Organ.

Liver Organ System

YANG PARTNER: Gallbladder
ELEMENT: Wood
SEASON: Spring
EMOTION: Patience, Kindness, Assertiveness, Aggression, Frustration, Anger
TASTE: Sour
COLOR: Green
TISSUE: Sinews, the tendons and ligaments
SENSE ORGAN: Eyes
GENERAL QUALITY: Gives us the ability to push through inertia, to grow, expand, and ultimately to "go with the flow."

The Liver and the Gallbladder belong to the Wood Element. Wood is the Element of beginnings, growth, and expansion. Spring is its season. The emergence of plants in the spring expresses the energy of the Wood Element.

The Liver is the Organ that keeps things growing, emerging, moving. The fresh bursting energy of spring is the landscape of the Liver.

Central concepts about the Liver

The Liver ensures the smooth flow of Qi throughout the meridian system.

The Liver keeps things moving. Blockages in the meridians create blockages in the flow of Qi, referred to as Qi stagnation. Qi backing up due to a block in a meridian is similar to traffic backing up behind a roadblock on a highway.

Liver energy imbues sprouts of springtime with what is needed to push through the heavy dirt above and reach for the Sun. Liver energy propels people forward and through any barrier. On a good day, this is called initiative, inspiration, motivation, and action. On a bad day, this energy is called frustration, anger, aggression, getting ahead regardless of the impact.

Picture the roadblock on the highway. On a bad day, as the traffic piles up, tempers flare. The more impatient and angry people get, the more aggressive they become trying to get around the stopped cars. As this energy increases we witness "fender benders" within the lines of traffic, and people yelling at each other.

On a good day, we chat with other drivers as we wait for the blockage to clear. Once the traffic begins to move again, people are polite and orderly, and we get on our way again easily and happily.

Spring is the season associated with the Liver Organ system. It is the beginning of Yang in the cycle of Yin and Yang through a year. This is the energy of new things, of birth and growth. Imagine the force it takes for plants to come out of the dormancy of winter to emerge upward again in the spring. Some of you know firsthand the force of giving birth. Liver energy is bursting outward and upward in the first stages of birth and growth.

Functions of the Liver

The Liver is in charge of keeping the Qi flowing smoothly. Like a steady overhead fan keeping the air moving, the Liver keeps the Qi moving. If it is too strong, a wind is created that agitates the entire system. If the Liver is overwhelmed and not functioning, Qi backs up in the meridians and energy is not supplied evenly throughout the body. As the Qi backs up we can feel frustrated and blocked, similar to being stopped in a traffic jam for too long.

Yang energy is protective of the more interior Yin. The Liver is very protective of our Life Force. Whenever we are threatened, our immediate defensive, reactive force comes from the Liver. This is the fight-or-flight aspect of the sympathetic nervous system. If we do not feel safe, our Liver energy is activated and ready to fight or run in order to save our life.

The Liver detoxifies the Blood at night while we sleep. Chinese medicine and Western medicine are similar in their understanding of the many detoxification processes associated with the Liver/liver. This important function is understood to happen while we rest at night. Therefore, if we are unable to sleep, we are unable to detoxify our Blood and our Liver gets overwhelmed and agitated. When this happens we tend to express frustration and anger rather than initiative and assertion.

Summary

The Liver needs space to grow and expand. When confined it feels hampered and blocked and will burst against that barrier. In human relationships this can look like one person yelling and screaming at the other who is "getting in the way" of one's hopes, dreams, or ambitions.

Spring is the time of youth and vigor. In the Western world, youth is highly valued even though we know it is a temporary stage of life. The attributes of the Liver—ambition, growth, external focus on other people, looking good (like new leaves on the trees in spring), movement, climbing up the corporate or social ladder—are emphasized as good and desirable in Western culture.

As a result the culture is very "Liver-like." Westerners partake of many external interventions to stay "springlike," such as stimulants, plastic surgery, excessive exercise, diets promising quick energy and youthful looks. Many diseases are now associated with "stress." From this perspective, stress can be seen as reacting to life events from the single focus of the Wood Element.

Western culture is so prone to believing that all things Liver are good—and everything else is bad, negative, or even frightening—that many of us have lost access to the resources of the other Elements and their qualities. The other Elements give us the resources that enable us to have a flexible, rather than reactive, response to the challenges and opportunities of our life.

Spring is certainly a wonderful time of the year and of life. Yet we all know that time moves on regardless of our desire to stay in one fixed place in the cycle. The ability to accept change and go with the flow requires access to all of our Organ systems. Being present in the moment and going with the flow are outward expressions of Qi moving and flowing along the meridian system. Being vibrant and happily going with the flow are manifestations of a balanced and content Liver Organ system.

Wood

Sprout

Anger / Kindness

Growing

Eyes

Tendons

Gallbladder

Spring

Wind

Liver

Heart Organ System

YANG PARTNER: Small Intestine

ELEMENT: Fire

SEASON: Summer

EMOTION: Joy, Love, Exuberance, Impatience, Over-excitement even Mania

TASTE: Bitter

COLOR: Red

TISSUE: Blood

SENSE ORGAN: Tongue

GENERAL QUALITY: Gives us the ability to communicate, to express our love and passion, to show off our creations.

Fire is the most Yang of the Five Elements. Fire is hot, flaming, rises up, captures our attention. In our world the Sun is our big Fire. The Sun lights up the entire world every day, shining light and warmth down onto the Earth. This massive Yang energy warms the Yin Earth. The Sun is the protective force of Yang that surrounds, lightens, and warms Earth.

The human equivalent of the Sun is the Heart Organ system. Our Heart is our light and warmth. The Heart is the Yin Organ of the most Yang Element, Fire.

Central concepts about the Heart

The Heart is home to our Spirit.

The Spirit is that energetic part of ourselves that resides in the physical body. The Spirit is Yang compared to the physical body which is Yin. To be alive is to have a Spirit residing in a body. At death, the body disintegrates, returning to the Earth, and the Spirit departs to return to the mysterious source of Nature. The Spirit is thought of as eternal, the body as temporary.

The Spirit is much greater than our personality, our thoughts and desires. The Spirit is difficult to describe but simple to appreciate. Consider who you really are, or who you have known yourself to be when you are at your very best, rising to the challenges of a difficult occasion. In these times, you act in virtuous ways beyond the usual modes of moodiness, judgment, or apathy. Your Spirit is the you that you know yourself to be that is not limited by your identity of name, job, personality, physical characteristics, reputation, relationships. This Spirit resides in your Heart.

If the Heart is agitated, the Spirit does not have a steady reliable place to reside. The Heart is agitated by too much celebration and exuberance, too much heat, too much extroversion, and too much mental or emotional stimulation. The Heart is depleted when there is no joy—too much cold, too much isolation, not enough stimulation. When the Heart is agitated or depleted, the Spirit is not secure in its home.

The manifestations of an insecure Spirit trying to reside in an agitated Heart are anxiety, mental restlessness, insomnia, and emotional instability. That may get so large as to lead to the bigger psychological conditions of delusions, psychosis, schizophrenia, etc.

Fire needs a root, a ground, a container. Without a root, Fire spreads and rises in every direction, unpredictably and dangerously. The root of Fire is Water, just as the root of Yang is Yin. The Kidneys are the Organs of the Water Element and will be discussed later on. Fire and Water are an essential Yang-Yin polarity within the body that everything else revolves around.

You may have been in the company of a very wise, warm, happy, quiet person. Their eyes sparkle, they are curious, present, attending to you and others, yet they abide fully within themselves. You are in the company of a quiet Heart that is home to a content Spirit.

You may have been in the company of a magnetic, energetic character who fills the room with a loud voice, jokes, and stories. Such people are the "life of the party," engaging with others, buzzing around the room, talking to everyone. After the party, they are exhausted and depressed. They don't know what they want or who they want to be. You are in the company of an agitated Heart and a confused Spirit.

Functions of the Heart

The Heart governs the Blood. Just as with the terms Organ/organ, the word Blood is capitalized when it indicates the Chinese medical term rather than the Western notion. It then refers to both the physical blood and the nourishing aspect of blood.

Blood is the tissue of the Heart. As repeated frequently in Chinese medicine: "Blood is the Mother of Qi and Qi is the Commander of Blood." This is a very important concept. Qi and Blood are a Yin-Yang pair. Qi needs a place to "be" as it is energetic, without material. Blood provides the material basis for the Qi, in the same way that the body provides the material basis for the Spirit. Blood needs a force to move and direct it. Qi is that force.

Without Blood there is no place for the Qi to reside or be nourished. Without Qi the Blood would not get pumped through the vessels nor would it stay within the vessels.

Summary

The Heart houses the Spirit, known as "Shen" in the Chinese language. The Heart governs the Blood, meaning that it provides the force for moving the Blood as well as the blood vessels which contain the Blood. The Heart thereby provides a home for our Spirit and our Qi (via the Blood). When the Heart is agitated, many psychological issues manifest.

火

Fire

Small Intestine

Sharing

Joy

San Jiao

Heat

Heart

Tongue

Showing

Summer

Flower

Hyper Extroversion

Blood

Pericardium Organ System

YANG PARTNER: San Jiao
ELEMENT: Fire
SEASON: Summer
EMOTION: Joy, Love, Exuberance, Impatience, Over-excitement even Mania
TASTE: Bitter
COLOR: Red
TISSUE: Blood
SENSE ORGAN: Tongue
GENERAL QUALITY: Gives us the ability to communicate, to express our love and passion, to show off our creations.

The Fire Element is the only Element that has four Organs: Heart, Small Intestine, Pericardium, San Jiao.

The Heart and Small Intestine are called "Cardinal Fire" (Big deal Fire) and the Pericardium and San Jiao are referred to as "Supplemental Fire" (not as big a deal as cardinal).

All of the Element associations are the same for the Pericardium as for the Heart, as shown in the list above.

The difference between Cardinal Fire and Supplemental Fire

Cardinal Fire is more like the big flame and Supplemental Fire is more like the low embers of a fire. Chinese medicine refers to the Heart Organ as the "Emperor." The Emperor is a very "Big Deal," in need of a large staff. All the other Organs can be considered as the staff of the Emperor. The Pericardium is the closest staff person to the Emperor.

Central concepts about the Pericardium

Pericardium is sometimes translated as "Heart Protector."

The pericardium is a sac around the heart and can easily be construed as a heart protector. Rather than speaking directly to the Emperor, you meet the Emperor's assistant, the Pericardium. This relationship is utilized in clinical practice by using Pericardium points and the meridian to treat the Heart.

In practice, there is not much of a distinction between the Heart and Pericardium. Some traditions never contact the Heart meridian in reverence to never directly touching the Emperor. In practice, points on the Pericardium meridian affect the Heart so they can be (and often are) used instead of Heart meridian points.

Functions of the Pericardium

Who we "open our heart to" has everything to do with the Pericardium. It is the Pericardium that holds the boundary around the Heart.

One way that hormones and opening our heart express in life is our sexual relationships. How we express ourselves sexually, who we open to, how we can connect from our heart, how we protect ourselves are all related to the Pericardium.

Summary

The Pericardium protects the Heart. It is the low level Fire, the more personal and intimate Fire relative to the big, more public, cardinal Fire expression of the Heart. Possibly the ancients' understanding of the complexity of love and our relationships is what guided them to putting four Organs within the Fire Element

Spleen Organ System

YANG PARTNER: Stomach
ELEMENT: Earth
SEASON: Late Summer
EMOTION: Satisfaction, Presence, Grounded, Worry
TASTE: Sweet
COLOR: Yellow
TISSUE: Muscle
SENSE ORGAN: Mouth and lips
GENERAL QUALITY: Gives us the ability to be a sturdy, safe, reliable presence. To give and receive nourishment, to manifest and enjoy our creations.

The Earth is our home. Everything grows out of the Earth. Our food grows in the Earth. The Earth provides a place and a home for everything we know. The muscles of our body give us our form, our physical mass, our home. All of the food we eat must be digested in order to extract its nutritive elements. Providing for the substances of our body, our "home," is the process of digestion and the central purpose of the Earth Element.

The Spleen is the Yin Organ of the Earth Element. In modern times the pancreas is associated with the Spleen and Earth Element.

Qi is a primary factor that is extracted during digestion. Every bodily function relies on Qi.

We gather Qi from our food, drink, and air. The Spleen is responsible for extracting Qi from food and drink. Qi acquired from digestion and breathing is referred to as post-Heaven Qi as we acquire it after our birth. If we are unable to extract Qi from our food, we will dip into our precious reserves of pre-Heaven Qi (discussed in Kidney section below) to fuel the body. Because our longevity depends on our pre-Heaven Qi we want to have plenty of post-Heaven Qi. It is essential that we supply our daily requirements of Qi with good food and great digestion, as this will conserve our pre-Heaven Qi and support our longevity.

When we have plenty of food, we are happy to share. When we have plenty of food, we feel satisfied at the end of our meal. Being satisfied on this level, we are relaxed and calm. Trusting in the abundance of our nutrition, we have a sense of safety and well-being. We are able to offer our help and support easily to others. When our physical body is satisfied and content, we are present within ourselves.

Having plenty of Qi, we have energy for our metabolism, strength for our daily activities and encounters with people and circumstances outside of ourselves. Our muscles have plenty of energy and so are supple, strong, and vital.

Central concepts about the Spleen

Digestion and Qi

To digest our food we must have a vital, happy Spleen.

Good digestion translates into plenty of Qi, which means plenty of energy and vitality. When digestion is impaired we do not get enough nutrition. When we are malnourished we spend our time looking for nutrition, worrying about not getting enough and eventually starving to death.

Our initial food came from our Mother. Mothers provide the actual physical basis for growing another human. Food, Mothers, Earth, and the Spleen are rolled up together in this perspective. A broader view of nutrition and digestion includes the ability to give and receive both physical and emotional nourishment, to digest the events of our lives, to feel the satisfaction of our efforts, to share our food, time, and expertise with others.

Functions of the Spleen

The Spleen must extract Qi from food through the process of digestion. The Qi that is extracted is sent up to the Lungs and Heart to be further transformed into "usable" Qi by the Lungs and then function as part of the process of making Blood in the Heart. Spleen Qi rises upward. Note that the Spleen plays an important part in the creation of Blood.

The quality and quantity of Blood is particularly important for women. Menstruating women lose Blood every month. Women who want to become pregnant require plentiful, vital Blood in order to maintain the health of their uterus.

Digestion is key to life no matter what medical perspective we use to look at it. In order to live we must eat and drink and be able to extract nutrition from our food. In Chinese medicine, the Spleen (along with the pancreas) is responsible for the digestive function of extracting nutrients, and most importantly, Qi.

Summary

The Spleen maintains digestive function and extracts Qi from food and drink. Qi is necessary for all of our functions, so the function of digestion is a central one in everyone's life. Plentiful food and a secure, reliable home contribute first to our sense of well-being, safety, and security, and then to our ease in sharing with and nourishing others. When these things are not in place, we feel worried, unsafe, unsatisfied, and without a sense of abundance. From this state we operate on scarcity, gathering more than we may need, hoarding, not sharing, and not having a sense of security and satisfaction.

Constant worry, circular ruminating, thinking about events out of our control—these inhibit the Spleen and thus digestion.

The Qi gathered by the Spleen during digestion is a key ingredient in making Blood.

Nutrition provides us with the substance to actually have a body, a home. Our first home was within our Mother's womb and she was physically responsible to nourish us. Mothering and all its attendant worries, responsibilities, and joys are linked with the Spleen and Earth Element.

Lung Organ System

YANG PARTNER: Large Intestine
ELEMENT: Metal
SEASON: Fall
EMOTION: Courage, Grief, Letting Go
TASTE: Pungent
COLOR: White
TISSUE: Skin
SENSE ORGAN: Nose
GENERAL QUALITY: Gives us the ability to feel ourselves, to have a boundary (skin), to contemplate inwardly, to let go of excess and keep the essential, to have courage of our convictions, to breathe.

Metal is the beginning of Yin in the cycle of the Five Elements. Fall is the season of Metal. The trees let go of their leaves, plants drop their seed and bring their sap or "energy" down into their roots. Letting go, going within, cooling off, and preparing for winter are activities of Fall.

The Lung Organ system performs these activities within the human being. Qi is often translated simply as "breath." The breath is within the Lung Organ system and therefore within the Metal Element. Meditation practices that bring stillness and reflection to the mind often focus on the breath. The ability to turn our attention inward, and the capacity for honest self-reflection, are resources of the Metal Element.

Fall and Spring are opposite seasons. Metal and Wood are opposite Elements. The opposing pairs balance one another. The outward expansion of Wood is tempered by the clarifying self-containment of Metal.

Central concepts about the Lung

The Lungs regulate and disseminate Qi.

Qi is what animates us. The concept of Qi is not present in Western culture, which makes it challenging to translate and to understand what the term refers to. Qi is often translated as "energy." Qi is also frequently translated as "breath."

The Lungs regulate and receive breath. We gather fresh Qi from the air with every inhalation and we release used-up Qi with every exhalation. The Spleen absorbs Qi from our food and water, the Lungs absorb Qi from the air we breathe. Without Qi we cannot live.

The depth, ease, and rhythm of our breath reflect the condition of our Body-Mind-Spirit. When we are in emotional upheaval our breathing is often rapid, out of control, shallow, and choppy. When we are deep in grief or sadness our breathing can feel heavy, exhausting, slow, and full of effort. When we are content in the moment, present with ourselves and our surroundings, our breath is rhythmical, easy, full, and delightful.

The practice of meditation focuses on the breath as a way of settling our minds and going inward. By consciously attending to our breath we become more aware of our true selves, our inner voice, mind and heart. The direction of going inward signifies the beginning of Yin in the cycle of the Five Elements. We learn to feel ourselves by feeling our breath and allowing our attention to be drawn inward, literally through the gateway of our breath. These qualities and characteristics are all associated with the Lungs and Metal Element.

When we say that the Lungs disseminate the Qi, we mean for one thing that they send the Qi downward and around the body. This Qi forms a protective layer called the Wei Qi, or Defensive Qi. I call this protective layer the "Qi jacket." Western medicine would refer to our healthy immune system. Regardless of the name, this Qi is what protects us from the external pathogens of the world (the weather conditions of cold, dry, hot, damp, wind). Just as the Heart pumps the Blood, the Lungs "pump" (disseminate) the Defensive (Wei) Qi around us, forming a protective layer of Qi.

In Chinese medicine the external pathogens are understood to invade our body where they can then enter into the meridian system and cause us harm. External pathogens can block the meridians, which interrupts the smooth flow of Qi in the meridian. Interrupting the smooth flow of Qi creates "Qi stagnation" that gives rise to physical manifestations such as pain, stuffy nose, headache, etc.

Most of us know that we should put on an extra layer of clothing or jacket when we go out into cold weather. We do this to prevent "getting a cold." Our built in, invisible coat is our "Qi jacket" or Defensive Qi. The "Qi jacket" prevents us from "catching a wind, heat, damp, or dry" in addition to the familiar "cold."

Prevention of illness is a hallmark of Chinese medicine and a primary intention of Meridian Massage. When the meridians have abundant, free-flowing Qi, external pathogens cannot enter and cause illness. Our Qi jacket, the first layer of protection from external pathogens, is a layer of Qi that circulates at the surface with the skin and protects us. By supporting the vitality of the Lung Organ system, we help keep our "Qi jacket" sturdy and zipped up.

The Lung Organ system includes the nose and respiratory system. Frequent colds are a clear sign that Lung Qi is low and the Defensive Qi is weak, allowing for pathogens to enter the meridian system.

Qi is acquired from the air we breathe.

In order to have plentiful Qi, our Lungs have to be in good shape. The Lungs and the Spleen are key Organs in the production of Qi. When there is fatigue, frequent colds or flus, allergies, or coughs there may be weakness in the Lungs and/or Spleen.

Functions of the Lungs

The Lungs are key to acquiring fresh Qi from the air and expelling used-up Qi during exhalation. The skin and Defensive (Wei) Qi are our first lines of defense from external pathogens. The Lungs are responsible for maintaining these defenses.

Fall is the season associated with the Lungs. Interestingly, this is known as "cold and flu" season in the West. Fall is also the time that the leaves are dropping and preparations are being made for winter. It is a time of letting go, reflection, contemplation, and inward attention. The Lungs support our ability to accept, decline, and move through our grief and losses that are a natural part of the cycle of life.

Summary

Breathing is vital to life. Qi is acquired when we breathe. Practices such as meditation, Qi Gong, and Tai Chi focus on the breath in order to build fresh Qi and clear out used Qi. This is similar to Western science's understanding that we inhale oxygen and exhale carbon dioxide.

Defending the body from external pathogens via the skin and Defensive Qi are responsibilities of the Lung Organ system.

Emotionally, the Lungs are related to grief, letting-go, and sadness. When we are overwhelmed by these emotions for too long, the Lungs may be injured, resulting in respiratory conditions such as cold, flu, or prolonged cough. You may have noticed that often people get a cold or flu shortly after the death of a loved one.

The emotion of courage, the qualities of self-reflection, and inward contemplation are also part of the Lung system. The Lungs give us the courage to face our situation and our feelings. By actively engaging with the events of our lifetime we are able to grow from them and gain wisdom over the years. This wisdom often comes in later life, in the "fall" of our life when we have wrinkled skin (the tissue of the Lung) and white (the color of the Metal Element) hair.

Self-reflection and contemplation are hardly recognized as valuable skills in our Western culture that values ambition, productivity, and extroversion above all else. The Lungs and Metal Element offer our stressed-out, overworked, tense, and frustrated culture a key to regaining balance and inner peace.

Metal

Large Intestine

Nose

Dry

Lung

Grief

Letting Go

Skin

Courage

Kidney Organ System

YANG PARTNER: Bladder
ELEMENT: Water
SEASON: Winter
EMOTION: Peace, Fear
TASTE: Salty
COLOR: Black or Blue
TISSUE: Bones
SENSE ORGAN: Ears
GENERAL QUALITY: Gives us the ability to create, to incubate and renew, to be a still and wise presence.

Water is the most Yin of the Five Elements. Here, in the hidden dark interior of the Kidneys, is our connection to the Source of our life, Kidney Essence. We receive the Essence of our life at the moment of conception—long before our awareness of ourselves is even formed. Long before we recognize the fact of our life, it has begun in the ancient, mysterious wonder of conception.

Yin is interior, inward, dark, and quiet, balancing Yang's external, outward, bright, loud expression. The Kidneys (Water) and Heart (Fire) are an essential polarity of Yin and Yang around which everything else revolves. The Essence gives the platform (a body) for the Spirit which resides in the Heart. The Heart gives expression to the immense potential of Life Force within the Essence.

Central concepts about the Kidney

The Kidneys hold our Life Force.

The Life Force being spoken of here is called "Jing," or Kidney Essence. Chinese medicine holds the Kidneys in high esteem as they are the containers of this precious Essence.

Pre-Heaven Essence

"Jing" or Kidney Essence is the "thing" that sustains us throughout our life. Pre-Heaven refers to before birth. We receive our pre-Heaven Essence from our biological parents at the moment of conception. The quantity and quality of this Essence will impact our entire life.

This Essence is very similar to the DNA in Western science, which says that our genes are inherited from our biological parents at the moment of conception. There is "nothing we can do about" the genes received at conception. They are the platform upon which our physical body is created.

Genes hold the codes to every molecule of all the cells that actually create our bodies. Growth, reproduction, constitutional tendencies, developmental factors, and timing are all under the "control" of our genes. Whether we will be tall or short, have blue eyes or green, are all unchangeable realities resulting from our genetic inheritance.

This notion of genes is similar to the Chinese notion of Essence. The Essence we receive is limited and unchangeable. It is our "constitution," what we have to work with in this lifetime.

It is said that when this pre-Heaven Essence runs out, so does our physical life. Therefore, longevity depends on conserving our pre-Heaven Essence. Conserving the pre-Heaven Essence means caring for our Kidneys.

We use our Essence to build Blood, Qi, and our physical body. We rely on post-Heaven Qi (absorbed and transformed by the Spleen and Lung) for our daily energy requirements. If we do not gather enough Qi from digestion and breathing, we will have to dip into our Essence to provide the missing energy. This is why Chinese medicine emphasizes lifestyle choices. We can conserve the Kidney Essence by eating well, breathing fresh air, getting adequate rest, and living in a way that supports our Spirit to feel peaceful, curious, and happy.

A simple prescription for a long happy healthy life—it's just not always so easy!

Functions of the Kidney

The Kidneys are responsible for growth, reproduction, and development.

These all depend on the vitality of our Kidneys. Any "issues," such as physical deformities, infertility, developmental delays, etc., reflect weak Kidney energy and specifically weak pre-Heaven Essence.

Kidneys hold our pre-Heaven Essence. Therefore, the key to longevity and health is preserving and maintaining the health of our Kidneys. The Kidneys are the Yin Organ of the Water Element, which is the most Yin Element in relationship to all of the other Elements. Yin is the ultimate nourishment for Yang. The basis for the flame (Fire, Yang) of a candle is the wax (Water, Yin).

The Kidneys provide the nourishing basis for all life as they are literally the holders of our Life Force. Although we tend to worship the flame, the wax provides the basis of that flame. Similarly, we tend to validate and celebrate Yang's expression, lightness, and voice while we ignore, forget, or even degrade

Yin's quiet, dark density. The Kidney Yin is nourished in the dark, in quiet, in sleep and stillness. When there is plentiful Yin, there can be plentiful Yang.

Summary

A long life relies on plenty of Essence. We use our Essence to build Blood, Qi, and our physical body. Essence is "lost" by men via semen. Women use Essence as the basis of creation during the development from zygote to baby in pregnancy. We all lose or use up Essence when we overexert our resources for extended amounts of time.

The Kidneys are most Yin of the Organs. They require rest, sleep, quiet, and calm in order to be restored and maintained. The Kidneys are the center of creation—both for physical reproduction and for creative endeavors. If our creativity is overdone or stunted, our Kidneys may be injured.

One way I think of Kidney Essence is as our "bounce back." When I was younger I could abuse myself often with hardly any ill effects. After a night of bad food and too much partying, I could still easily bounce back the next day. Fast forward thirty years: If I eat too much ice cream after dinner, I really feel it the next morning. This is a sign that my bounce back is depleted—which is a nice way of saying that I'm older and now have less Kidney Essence than I did thirty years ago.

Most people have a list in their heads of the things they know to do or not do in order to be "healthy." These are lifestyle choices. From this perspective, the reason to be mindful of our daily choices is to preserve our precious Kidney Essence so that we live a long and happy life.

Water

Store

Incubating

Winter

Cold

Ear

Bladder

Part 2

Tools of the Trade

1: Twelve Meridians

The Twelve Meridians and their Key Points

Just as the riverbed is where the water of the river flows, meridians are where the Qi flows. Meridians are not seen and are not physical structures, yet they are real and present in every body. They run lengthwise along the limbs, trunk, and head in channels that were mapped out ages ago.

There are twelve "regular" meridians. Each named meridian is located on both limbs or sides of the body, although the diagrams that illustrate the text here only show them on one limb or side. Named points on meridians are likewise located on both limbs and both sides of the body in the corresponding places left and right.

Meridian Massage utilizes contact to meridians and points (also known as acupoints) to support the harmonious flow of Qi throughout the network of meridians.

How to Use the Following Pages

Every meridian is described in a number of ways including whether it is a Yin or Yang meridian and its association within the Five Element perspective and Six Channel perspective. The Six Channel perspective is less familiar for many people and is discussed separately in Chapter 3 here in Part 2. I provide a reference page for each meridian and the key points for the meridian that you can return to as you continue your studies. All meridians and points are located on both sides and limbs of the body. The diagrams show only one side so that the student can visualize the pathway or point on the other side.

Point Combinations

In practice many points are used in combination with one another to achieve a desired result. There are many ancient point combinations that are so effective that they have been handed down for thousands of years. I list some of the more common combinations where applicable. For more information on these combinations, see Part 2, Chapter 8.

Point Categories

Certain points belong to special categories. For example, there is a set of points known as "Command Points." For each area of the body—neck, abdomen, back, etc.—there is a certain acupoint that is the Command Point of that area. When needed, we use Command Points to help direct the flow of Qi to this area during the session.

Points that belong to certain categories are so noted in this text. Of the many point categories, I include Command Points, Ma Dan Yang's Heavenly Star Points, Master Points of the extraordinary vessels, and Yuan Source Points, which are discussed in Chapters 4–7 of Part 2.

Point Names and Numbers

Points were given names in ancient times. These names give clues as to the location and/or action(s) of the point. When Chinese medicine was exported, the points were numbered to make them easier for Westerners to learn. For visual clarity, the images in this text use only the number; the names are given in the explanations.

There are hundreds of points on the twelve regular meridians. This text identifies and gives uses for 108 points: 96 of the points on the twelve regular meridians and twelve points on the Du and Ren (extraordinary vessels). These points are relevant to the practice of Meridian Massage. Rest assured that learning this set of points will serve you and your clients well for years to come!

Point Location Essentials

Point locations are based on precise measurements from visible landmarks. The distances given are referred to as cun ("tsoon"). One cun is measured by the width of a thumb (see diagrams). Because body size varies, one cun on my body will be a different size than one cun on your body.

Cun measurements are proportional to each body. Early practitioners discovered these relational distances and used them to describe point location. This book follows in that tradition of directing the reader to the point using cun measurements. The diagrams below show how the body is measured by cuns.

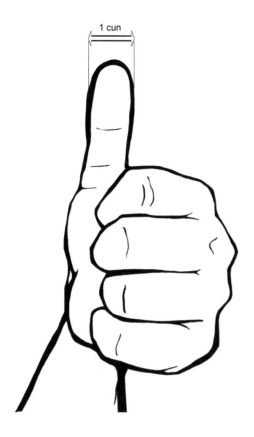

1 cun

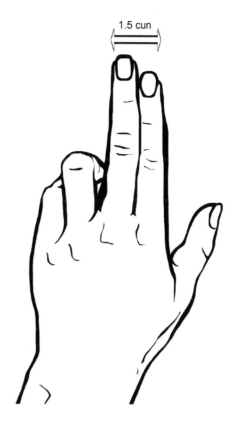

1.5 cun

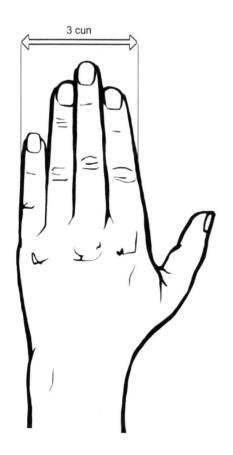

3 cun

When locating points on another person, first note the relative size difference between your hand, fingers, and thumbs and theirs. You will adjust distances that you measure on another person based on the relative size difference between your bodies.

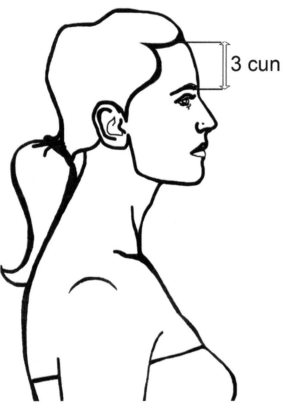

3 cun

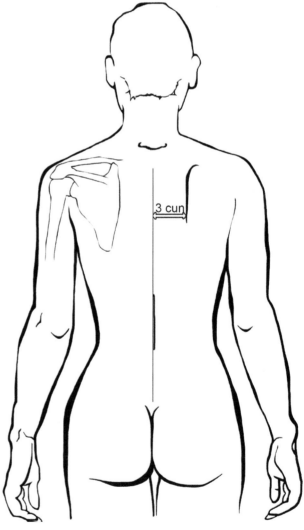

3 cun

Using the cun proportions here and on page 85 is more precise than using thumbs or fingers on another person. The proportions shown are relative to each person. For example, the Bladder meridian line is 1.5 cun from the spine. Note that from the spine to the medial border of the scapula (shoulder blade) is 3 cun. Regardless of the person's size, 1.5 cun from their spine is halfway between the spine and the medial border of the scapula.

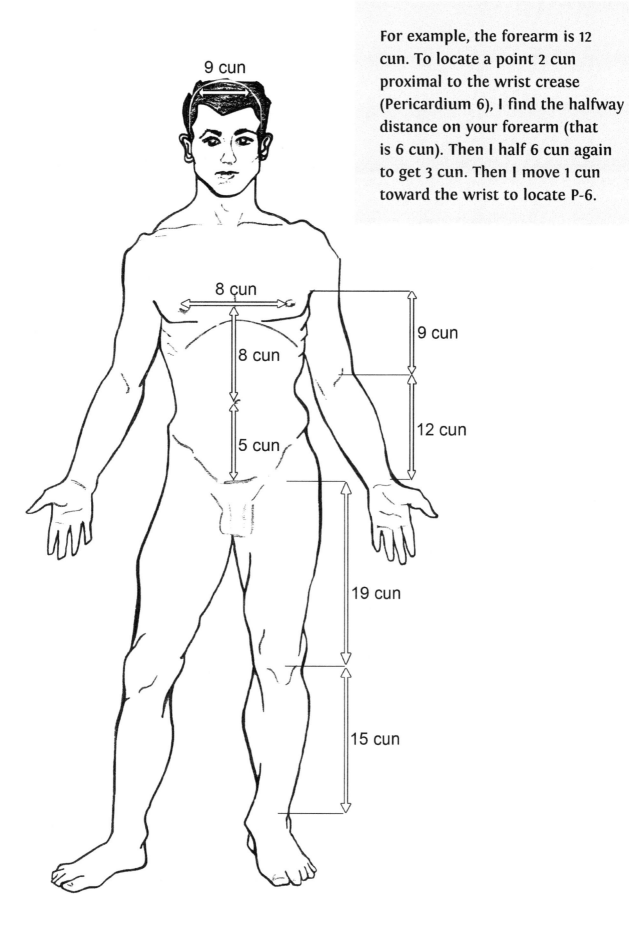

9 cun

8 cun

8 cun

5 cun

9 cun

12 cun

19 cun

15 cun

For example, the forearm is 12 cun. To locate a point 2 cun proximal to the wrist crease (Pericardium 6), I find the halfway distance on your forearm (that is 6 cun). Then I half 6 cun again to get 3 cun. Then I move 1 cun toward the wrist to locate P-6.

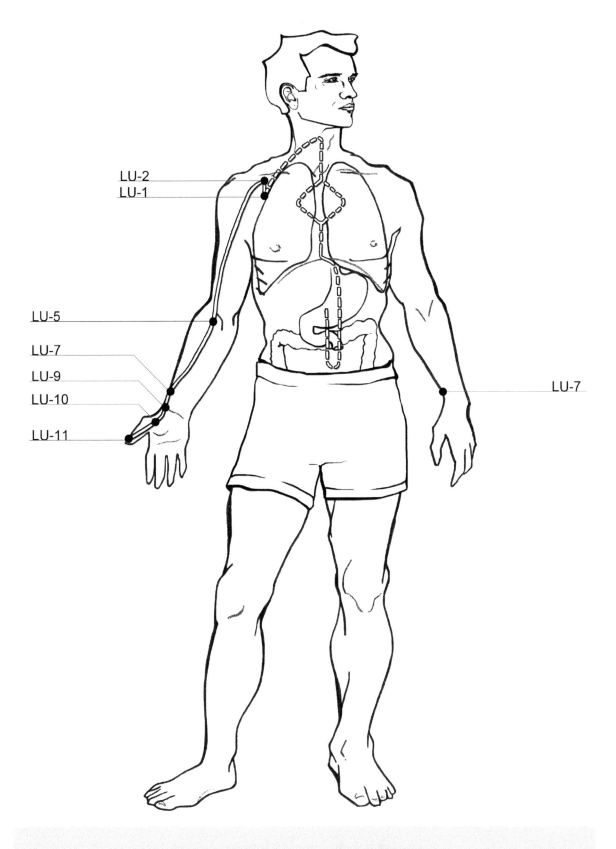

LU-2
LU-1

LU-5

LU-7

LU-9

LU-10

LU-11

LU-7

LUNG MERIDIAN | HAND TAI YIN

Lung Meridian

Yin

Five Element perspective
Element: Metal
Yang partner: Large Intestine

Six Channel perspective
Lung channel of the hand Tai Yin (Greatest Yin)
Paired with: Spleen channel of the foot Tai Yin (Greatest Yin)

Key points: LU-1, 2, 5, 7, 9, 10

Beginning point: LU-1 on the chest a few inches below the lateral end of the clavicle

End point: LU-11 on the thumb

The Lung meridian is one of three Yin meridians on the upper part of the body. Yin meridians are located on the anterior (front), Yin, surfaces. On the arm, this surface is the anterior forearm (same surface as the palm) and the anterior upper arm where the biceps are located (see diagram #).

External pathway

This meridian comes to the surface at LU-1 on the chest. It crosses the anterior shoulder and runs down the lateral edge of the anterior (front) surface of the upper arm and ends on the thumb. The meridian is lateral to the biceps muscle, crosses the anterior elbow (lateral to the biceps tendon), continues on the lateral edge of the anterior forearm, crosses the wrist to run along the palmar side of first metatarsal up the side of the thumb, and ends at LU-11 on the lateral nail base of the thumbnail.

Internal pathway

The internal pathway creates a connection between the paired Metal Organs, Lung and Large Intestine. The internal pathway also helps to explain how LU-10 has an effect on the throat. The interior Lung meridian begins in the stomach, drops to the large intestine, makes its way up through the diaphragm and lungs, up into the throat, and then back down to emerge at LU-1.

Think of the Lung meridian when:

Any respiratory condition arises or persists.
Any breathing issues arise or persist.
Fatigue is chronic.

Approaching the Lung Meridian

As it is a Yin Organ, we want to nourish, tonify, build up the Lung. Even when there is a respiratory condition such as a cold or flu, we are gentle with the Lung. Use the Large Intestine (Lung's Yang partner) to more vigorously move Qi and clear away pathogens in the event of a cold or flu.

Check the breathing rate and depth. Consider working on the abdomen and diaphragm in order to create more space for the lungs to expand upon inhalation. Be sensitive to the emotion of grief that can come to the surface and release as the breath deepens and the person allows themself to feel their lungs.

The Lung is a key player in transforming and spreading Qi. The air we breathe contains Qi. Fatigue is a sign of lack of Qi. Since air is a direct source of Qi, lack of Qi and energy (fatigue) directs us, in part, to the Lung. (The Spleen is another big player in the acquisition of Qi.)

Lung Points (LU-1, 2, 5, 7, 9, 10)

Lung 1: Zhong Fu, "Middle Palace"

Location: Inferior to the lateral clavicle, 6 cun lateral to the midline, 1 cun inferior to LU-2.
Location tip: LU-1 is at the first intercostal space, on the rib cage. Be sure your pressure is toward the ribs rather than the arm.

Use:
To open the Lungs, open the rib cage, and support the breath
To relieve respiratory conditions

Lung 2: Yun Men, "Cloud Gate"

Location: Inferior to the lateral clavicle, 1 cun superior to LU-1.
Location tip: LU-2 is the large dip created in the deltoid-pectoral muscles when flexing the shoulder (bringing the arm straight out in front).

Use:

To open the Lungs, open the rib cage, and support the breath

To relieve respiratory conditions

To relieve local shoulder pain

Lung 5: Chi Ze, "Cubit Marsh"

Location: In the anterior elbow crease just lateral to the biceps tendon.

Location tip: Bend the elbow and clearly feel the biceps tendon. The hollow just lateral (on the thumb side) to the tendon is LU-5.

Use:

For local elbow pain

To clear phlegm from the lungs

Lung 7: Lie Que, "Broken Sequence"

Location: Just proximal to the styloid process of the radius, between the tendons of brachioradialis and abductor pollicis longus.

Location tip: Gently place a finger on the thumb side of the radial styloid process and slide proximally, feeling for a dip between the two tendons.

Use:

LU-7 is:

1) The Command Point of the neck [12] —use it when there are any neck issues.

2) The Master Point of the Ren [13]

3) It opens the Ren vessel [14]

4) One of Ma Dan Yang's Heavenly Star Points [15]

Use this point to relieve symptoms of colds and flus, to support and nourish the Lungs and the Metal Element.

Point combination:

LU-7 + KD-6 is a Master Point [16] combination that is deeply nourishing for the Yin energy throughout the body. Using it brings calm, quiet, and stillness to the entire body-mind.

Lung 9: Tai Yuan, "Great Abyss"

Location: On the radial (thumb side) edge of the anterior wrist crease.

Location tip: Find the wrist pulse then slide toward the hand and feel for the large dip at the wrist crease.

LU-9 is the Yuan Source Point [17] of the Lung meridian.

Use:
To nourish the Lungs, especially during long-term illness such as pneumonia or chronic obstructive pulmonary disorder

Lung 10: Yu Ji, "Fish Border"

Location: On the thenar eminence, at the midpoint of the first metacarpal, on the palmar aspect.
Location tip: Find the midpoint of the first metacarpal and feel for the dip on the thenar side of the bone.

Use:
For local pain and to support the health of local circulation and muscles
To relieve sore throat

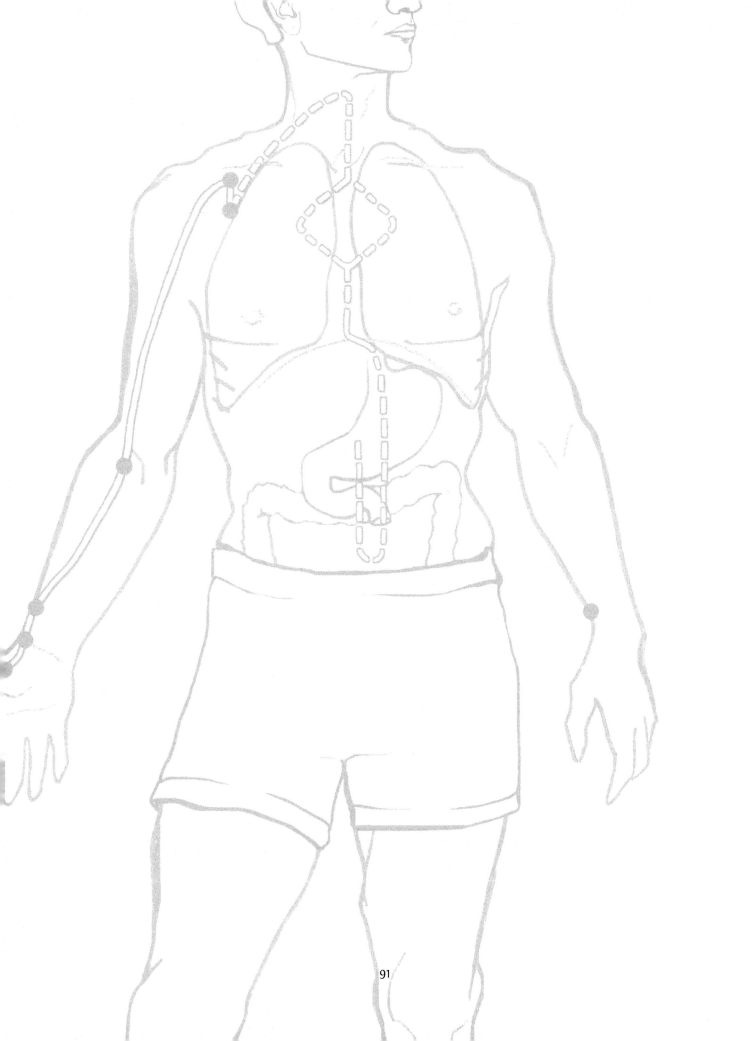

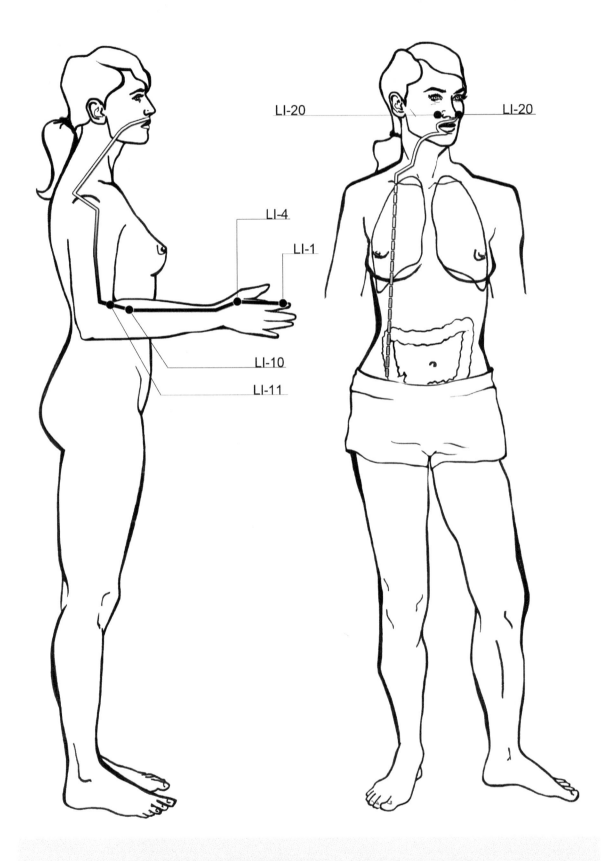

LI-20

LI-20

LI-4

LI-1

LI-10

LI-11

LARGE INTESTINE MERIDIAN | HAND YANG MING

Large Intestine Meridian

Yang

Five Element perspective
Element: Metal
Yin partner: Lung

Six Channel perspective
Large Intestine channel of the hand Yang Ming
Paired with Stomach channel of the foot Yang Ming

Key points: LI-4, 10, 11, 20

Beginning point: LI-1 on the lateral nail bed of first finger

End point: LI-20, next to the nostril

External pathway

The Large Intestine is one of three Yang meridians on the upper arm. Yang meridians are located on the posterior, Yang (back) surface of the body. On the arm, this surface is the posterior forearm (same surface as the back of the hand and the posterior upper arm where the triceps are located).

Notice that LU-11 is on the thumb. Qi flows through the twelve meridians in an orderly fashion. From the Lungs, the next meridian is the LI (Large Intestine). Qi moves from the thumb (LU-11—the last point of the Lung meridian) to the first finger (LI-1).

From LI-1, the external pathway of the Large Intestine meridian moves along the "thumb side" of the first finger, through the web of the thumb and first finger, through the anatomical "snuff box" and along the lateral edge of the posterior surface of the forearm and upper arm. The meridian crosses the lateral aspect of the shoulder, over the acromion process to the lateral aspect of the neck, up to the jaw, cheeks, and ends at the edge of the opposite nostril (LI-20).

Internal pathway

The interior Large Intestine meridian begins at the Stomach meridian point ST-12, located at the midpoint of the clavicle. The Large Intestine meridian "dives" internally from this point and connects with the lungs, goes through the diaphragm to connect to the large intestine.

Think of the Large Intestine meridian when:

There is pain in the head, face, teeth, shoulder, forearm, hand (along the path of the meridian).
There is any respiratory condition.
There is too much heat, as in a fever, hot flashes, high blood pressure, anxiety, hot temper, hyperactivity.
Dealing with grief, loss, letting go, endings, Fall.

Approaching the Large Intestine meridian

Because it is a channel for a Yang Organ, we can use this meridian to vigorously move Qi and clear away the pathogens. Pain along the meridian is common, for example tennis elbow (LI-10, 11) and shoulder pain. Pain often arises from Qi stagnation. It is generally more common to see these issues arise along Yang meridians than Yin meridians. Yang Qi is active, forceful, moving. Apply more movement, shaking, stretching, and bouncing to get the Qi moving in the Yang meridians.

Check the breathing rate and depth. Consider working directly on the large intestine to encourage peristalsis, relaxation, and ease in the intestines. On inhalation, the lungs expand and the diaphragm descends to the abdominal cavity (well, it has that potential). Stagnation of Qi, emotions, and waste in the intestines can limit the downward motion of the diaphragm, thus limiting the breath.

By massaging the large intestine, we create space for deep breathing. Be sensitive to the emotion of grief (and other emotions) that can come to the surface and release as the breath deepens and awareness connects with the abdomen.

Large Intestine points (4, 10, 11, 20)

LI-4: He Gu, "Joining Valley"

Location: In the web between the thumb and first finger, dorsal surface.
Location tip: Adduct (bring the thumb next to first finger) the thumb so that you see a crease where the web was. Notice the high point on the finger side of the proximal crease—that is LI-4. Hold pressure and open the thumb.

LI-4 is:
1) The Command Point of the face and head—Use it when there are any face or head issues.
2) One of Ma Dan Yang's Heavenly Star Points.
3) The Yuan Source Point of the Large Intestine.

Use:*
LI-4 is the Command Point of the face and head. Use it for any symptoms of head or face.
It is a key point for headaches, toothache, congestion or cough from colds, flus, and any painful conditions of the head.

It is an important point for all respiratory conditions (Yang pair of the Lung Meridian).
*Use of this point is contra-indicated in pregnancy, as it induces labor.

Point combination:
LI-4 + LV-3 is referred to as "Four Gates." This combination opens the flow of Qi throughout the body.

LI-10: Shou San Li, "Arm Three Miles"

Location: 2 cun distal to LI-11 on the brachioradialis.
Location tip: With the elbow flexed and forearm in "neutral," find LI-11 then slide distally 2 cun to LI-10.

Use:
For local pain, tennis elbow. Notice that LI-10 mirrors the location (and name) of Stomach meridian ST-36 on the leg.

Point combination:
LI-10 + ST-36 to support immune system

LI-11: Qu Chi, "Pool at the Crook"

Location: At the tip of the lateral crease of the elbow.
Location tip: Flex the elbow and locate the point at the lateral tip of the crease. Pressure is directed toward the medial elbow.

LI-11 is one of Ma Dan Yang's Heavenly Star Points.

Use:
To clear heat (fever, high blood pressure, hyperactivity, red/dry conditions of the skin, anger)—this is a very important point for clearing heat!
For local pain, tennis elbow

LI-20: Ying Xiang, "Welcome Fragrance"

Location: At the base of the nostril.
Location tip: Place finger at side of left nostril, slide down into the dip of LI-20.

Use:
To open the nose and sinuses and clear congestion

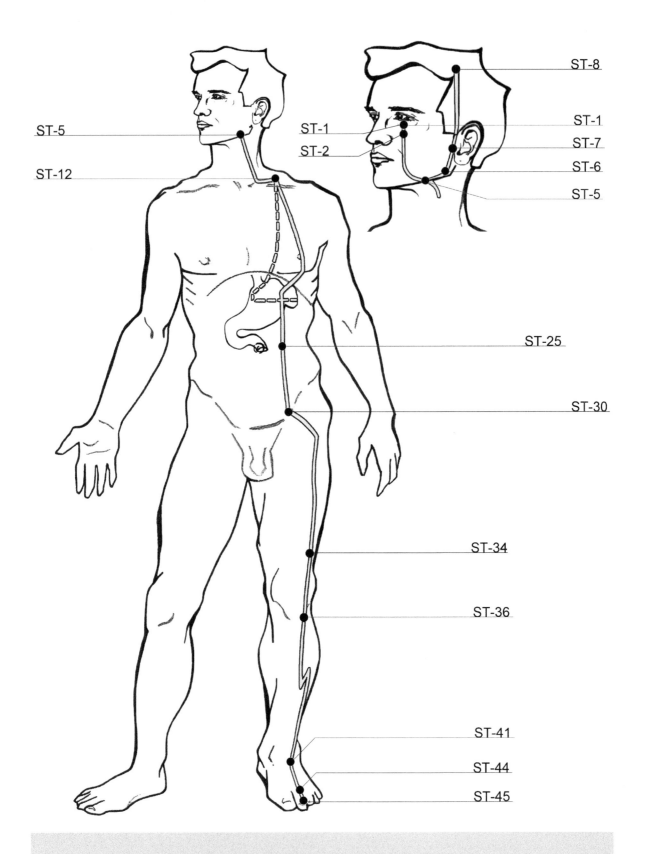

ST-5

ST-12

ST-1
ST-2

ST-8

ST-1
ST-7
ST-6
ST-5

ST-25

ST-30

ST-34

ST-36

ST-41
ST-44
ST-45

STOMACH MERIDIAN | FOOT YANG MING

Stomach Meridian

Yang

Five Element perspective
Element: Earth
Yin partner: Spleen

Six Channel perspective
Stomach channel of the foot Yang Ming
Partnered with Large Intestine channel of the hand Yang Ming

Key points: ST-2, 5, 6, 7, 12, 25, 34, 36, 41, 44

Beginning point: ST-1 directly below the pupil on the infraorbital ridge

Ending point: ST-45 on the lateral nail bed of the second toe

External pathway

The Stomach meridian is the only Yang meridian located on the anterior, Yin, surface of the body. It begins just below the eyeball, on the inferior rim of the orbital ridge, at ST-1. The meridian drops down to the jaw, then goes back up the side of the head and descends again via the anterior-lateral aspect of the neck, runs down the ribs (passing through the nipple), across the abdomen and anterior hip to the lateral aspect of the quadriceps, along the lateral edge of the patella, descends just lateral to the tibia, across the anterior ankle, and ends on the second toe at ST-45.

Note that although the meridian is anterior, it is on the lateral (Yang) aspect of the leg.

Internal pathway

The internal branch descends from ST-12 (located at the midpoint of the clavicle) through the diaphragm and connects with the stomach and spleen.

Think of the Stomach meridian when:

This is a very long meridian so it is used for symptoms from head to toe. Use it for:
Any digestive issues, stomach ulcers, hiatal hernia, acid indigestion, constipation, diarrhea, spastic colon.
Toothaches, abscesses, gum issues, lip conditions.
Any pain along the pathway of the meridian.
Eating issues or disorders.

Approaching the Stomach meridian

The Stomach and Spleen are the Organs of the Earth Element. Digestion is key to our health. We replenish our Qi by eating good food, drinking healthy liquids, and breathing fresh air. This daily replenishment is our post-Heaven (after birth) Qi. Our relationship to nutrition is entwined with the Stomach.

If we are unable to replenish our stock of Qi daily, we will reach into our stock of pre-Heaven Essence (what we received at conception) to support the functions of our body, mind, and spirit. We live as long as we have pre-Heaven Essence. So a long life is dependent on preserving our pre-Heaven Essence and replenishing our post-Heaven Qi every day. The Earth Element is a key player in digesting and absorbing food and fluids needed for our daily Qi supply.

When we eat or drink, the food must go down. After we absorb the Qi through digesting, Qi must be sent upwards to the chest and head, and out to all of the extremities.

Within the Earth Element, the Stomach is responsible for the downward flow of energy, and the Spleen is responsible for the upward flow. The Spleen transports Qi and fluids up (to the chest and brain) and out to the limbs. The Stomach keeps the flow of food and waste going down.

The Stomach meridian is a Yang meridian, so we can use more vigor and movement in our massage. Digestive issues will inevitably entail massage to the abdomen. Working the Stomach meridian on the lower leg before going to the abdomen creates more ease and readiness for the abdominal massage.

Stomach Points (ST-2, 5, 6, 7, 12, 25, 34, 36, 41, 44)

ST-2: Si Bai, "Four Whites"

Location: 1 cun below the iris in the infraorbital foramen.
Location tip: With your client's eyes open and looking straight ahead, locate ST-2 directly below the iris on the zygomatic bone that forms the lower eye socket. The infraorbital foramen feels like a little hole or dip in the bone. ST-2 is one cun below the eye.

Use:
To relieve eye strain or fatigue
To relieve pain from sinus congestion

ST-5: Da Ying, "Great Welcome"

Location: Just anterior to the angle of the mandible in the dip next to the border of the masseter muscle.

Location tip: Place finger on the chin and slide along the jaw until you bump into the lower attachment of the masseter muscle just before the angle of the mandible. ST-5 is in the dip on the mandible at the border of this muscle. ST-6 is in the muscle belly. ST-5 is on the jaw bone not the masseter muscle.

Use:
For jaw pain, tooth pain

ST-6: Jia Che, "Jaw Bone"

Location: On the angle of the mandible in the dip in the center of the lower attachment of the masseter muscle.
Location tip: Place finger on the jaw and slide laterally until you bump into the lower attachment of the masseter muscle, keep going to feel the muscle attachment bundle and find the dip which is ST-6.
Note: ST-5 is on the mandible (jaw bone) next to the masseter bone, ST-6 is in the center of the lower attachment of the masseter muscle.

Use:
For jaw pain, tooth pain, tight jaw

ST-7: Xia Guan, "Below the Joint"

Location: Anterior to the ear, below the zygomatic arch.
Location tip: Place finger on the condyle of the mandible, just below the zygomatic arch. Ask the client to open their mouth, and feel the condyle bulge beneath your finger. When they close their mouth you will feel the depression which is the point.

Use:
For TMJ syndrome, jaw tension
For ear pain, infection, stuffiness, tinnitus
For teeth pain

ST-12: Que Pen, "Empty Basin"

Location: Superior to the midpoint of the clavicle.
Location tip: Find the center of the clavicle and roll your pressure gently into the tender tissue of the neck region.

Use:
This is the meeting point of all of the Yang meridians of the arm, the Gallbladder and Stomach meridians. It is an important point for opening the chest, so that descending Lung Qi flows smoothly.

ST-25: Tian Shu, "Heaven's Pivot"

Location: Two cun lateral to the navel.
Location tip: This is the midpoint (from lateral to medial) of the rectus abdominus ("six-pack") muscle.

Use:
For digestive complaints

Point combination:
ST-25 + ST-36 to relieve digestive complaints.

ST-34: Liang Qiu, "Ridge Mound"

Location: 2 cun proximal (toward the hip) of the upper border of the patella.
Location tip: Use the lateral border of the patella as your guide, slide your pressure up from the patella 2 cun and feel for a dip in the quadriceps.

Use:
For acute stomach pain or upset

ST-36: Zu San Li, "Leg Three Miles"

Location: 3 cun inferior to the lower tip of patella, one thumb width lateral to tibia.
Location tip: Locate the tibial tuberosity and go one thumb width lateral to the tibia. This point is in the tibialis anterior muscle.

ST-36 is:
1) Command Point of the abdomen
2) One of Ma Dan Yang's Heavenly Star Points

Use:
This is an extremely powerful point for building the resources of the body. Use it
For all abdominal issues, and specifically for digestive concerns.
To build Qi and Blood

Point combinations:
ST-36 + LI-10—to support the immune system.
ST-36 + SP-6—to build Blood. This is very good for menstruating women.
ST-36 + ST-25—for digestive complaints.

ST-41: Jie Xi, "Stream Divide"

Location: Anterior ankle between the two malleoli, in the depression between the tendons of extensor hallucis longus and extensor digitorum longus.

Location tip: Sink pressure just lateral to the tibialis anterior tendon as it crosses the anterior ankle. ST-41 is in the center of the "front," anterior, ankle.

Use:

To open the ankle (draws Qi down the meridian, opens the leg)
For local pain and pain in the upper reaches of the meridian

ST-44: Nei Ting, "Inner Courtyard"

Location: Dorsal surface of the foot, at the junction between the second and third toes.

Location tip: Place a finger between the second and third toe and slide toward the ankle just .5 cun.

Use:

ST-44 clears Fire-Heat from the Stomach meridian, so use it for:

Stomach ulcers

Tooth abscesses

Indigestion

Acid reflux

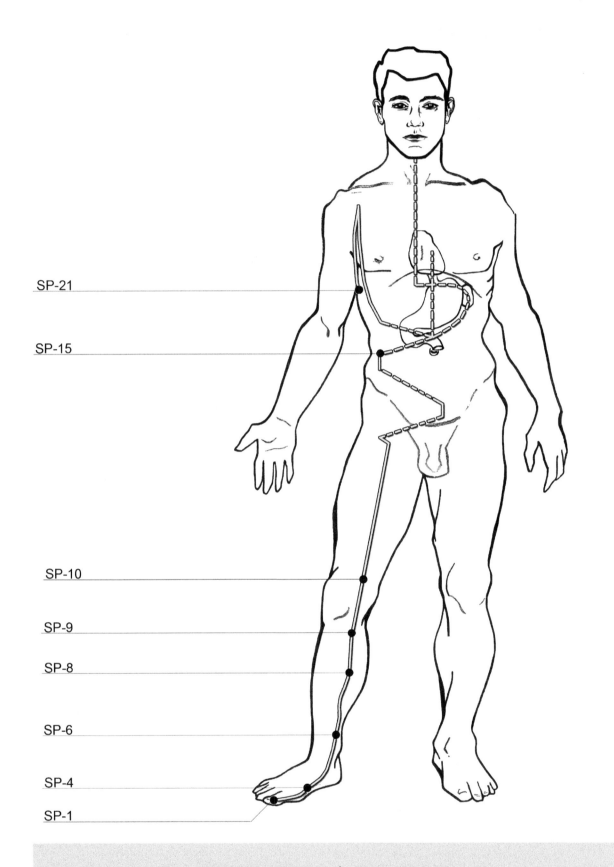

SP-21

SP-15

SP-10

SP-9

SP-8

SP-6

SP-4

SP-1

SPLEEN MERIDIAN | FOOT TAI YIN

Spleen Meridian

Yin

Five Element perspective
Element: Earth
Yang partner: Stomach

Six Channel perspective
Spleen channel of the foot Tai Yin
Partnered with Lung channel of the hand Tai Yin

Key points: SP-4, 6, 8, 9, 10, 15

Beginning point: SP-1 on the medial nail bed of the big toe

End point: SP-21 on the lateral border of the rib cage between seventh and eighth rib

External pathway

This is a Yin meridian, so it will be on the inner leg surface, on the abdomen and ribs. This is the most anterior of the Yin meridians of the leg.

The Spleen meridian begins at SP-1, located on the medial corner of the nail bed of the big toe. It runs along the arch of the foot, comes up the anterior edge of the medial malleolus then up the medial leg, medial edge of the patella, medial border of the quadriceps, up to the abdomen (four cun lateral to the navel), up the ribs (lateral to the breast), up to the armpit area, and then drops down to end on the lateral rib cage in the space between the seventh and eighth ribs at SP-21.

Internal pathway

When the Spleen meridian reaches the inguinal area, it dives internally and connects with some REN points, then goes back to external Spleen points on the abdomen. This forms a zigzag pattern from REN to SP to REN to SP. From REN-12, the meridian begins its internal pathway where it connects with spleen, stomach, and heart and then rises up to end at the base of the tongue.

Think of the Spleen meridian when:

There are any digestive issues.
There is fatigue, weakness in the limbs.
There is heaviness, fogginess, lethargy, inertia.
There are Blood issues: heavy or scanty menstruation, anemia, varicose veins, easy or excess bruising.
There are fertility issues.

Approaching the Spleen meridian

In women, this meridian and its points are often tender, so apply pressure gradually.
The Earth Element contains all aspects of our nourishment. Consider the Earth to literally be the Mother. Mothers are where every person first came into being and grew into our human form. We relied on our Mothers as embryos and fetuses. As infants we completely rely on our Mothers for nourishment (milk), protection, and stability.

The Spleen is the Yin Organ of the Earth Element, and as such it is the center of nourishment and all things having to do with mothering, mothers, fertility, menstruation, eating, digesting, and absorbing. The source of our food, of our substance, is Earth. Within the human microcosm, we grow ourselves physically from the food we eat. Every cell must receive Qi and Blood. That Qi and Blood rely on nutrition, digestion, and absorption in order to be created within the body in the first place. This shows us the connection between the Spleen and the Stomach to the general energy (Qi) level, our physical strength and form, muscle mass, fertility, quality of blood, and our general sense of being present or available. It also connects with our generosity—the Earth gives of itself in order to create us, just as our Mother shared her nutrition, air, blood, and minerals with us in the womb.

Spleen Points (SP-4, 6, 8, 9, 10, 15)

SP-4: Gong Sun, "Grandfather Grandson"

Location: On the arch of the foot, just distal to the tibialis anterior tendon.
Location tip: Place a finger on the arch of the foot near the big toe. Have the client invert and dorsiflex their foot and you will see the tibialis anterior tendon clearly. Slide along the arch and feel for the dip of SP-4. (SP-4 is distal to this tendon, KD-2 is proximal to it.)

SP-4 is a Master Point of the Chong extraordinary vessel.[18] Use it:
To open, stimulate the Chong (which is very important to Blood and the uterus in women)
To support the Spleen

Point combination:

SP-4 + P-6 to settle the interior, stimulate parasympathetic rest and digest, calm the heart. (Master Point combination.)

SP-6: San Yin Jiao, "Three Yin Meeting"

Location: 3 cun proximal to the high point of the medial malleolus.
Location tip: Place your pinky on the high point of the medial malleolus—the border of your first finger is the 3 cun measurement. The point is midway between the anterior and posterior edges of the leg.

Use:*
As the name implies, the three Yin meridians of the leg meet at SP-6, so this is a key point for nourishing the Liver, Kidney, and Spleen. This point is often very tender on women, so increase pressure gradually. Use it
To nourish Blood
To support the consistent rhythm of the menstrual cycle
To relieve menstrual cramps
*Contra-indicated in pregnancy

Point combination:
SP-6 + ST-36 to build Qi and Blood.

SP-8: Di Ji, "Earth Pivot"

Location: 3 cun distal to SP-9.
Location tip: Measure 3 cun distal from SP-9 using a hand width.

Use:
For acute menstrual cramps.
This point is often very tender on women, so increase pressure gradually.

SP-9: Yin Ling Quan, "Yin Mound Spring"

Location: On the medial leg just below the tibial condyle.
Location tip: Gently glide your finger up the medial border of the tibia. Where it turns, move into the flesh and feel for the point.

Use:
To drain Damp. Use when there is general puffiness from humid weather, excess weight, foggy thinking, sluggish digestion due to the Spleen being weakened from Dampness.

SP-10: Xue Hai, "Sea of Blood"

Location: On the medial thigh, 2 cun proximal to the upper border of the patella.
Location tip: The Spleen meridian is in line with the medial border of the patella. Glide proximally along the medial border of patella and 2 cun superior to the top of the patella, feel for the dip of SP-10.

Use:
To clear toxins from the blood
To help clear drugs, medications, chemotherapy from blood

SP-15, Da Heng, "Great Horizontal"

Location: 4 cun lateral to the navel.
Location tip: This point is on the same level as ST-25 (see p. 96) at the lateral border of rectus abdominis.

Use:
For digestive complaints

Point combinations:
ST-36 + ST-25 + SP-15 to relieve digestive complaints.

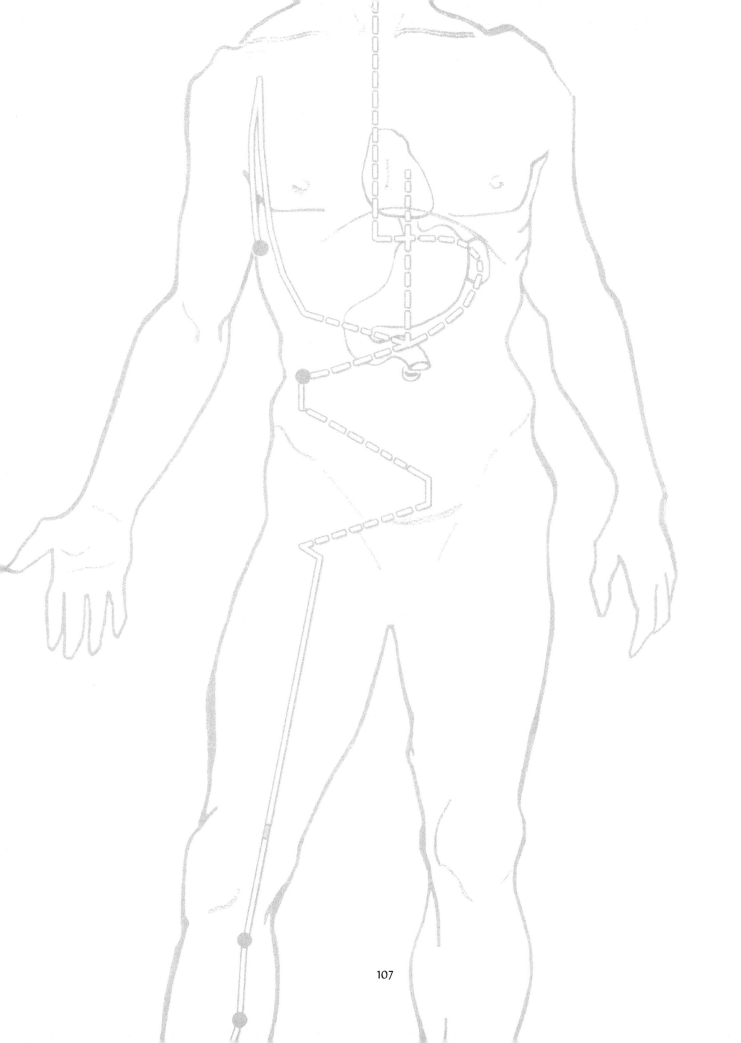

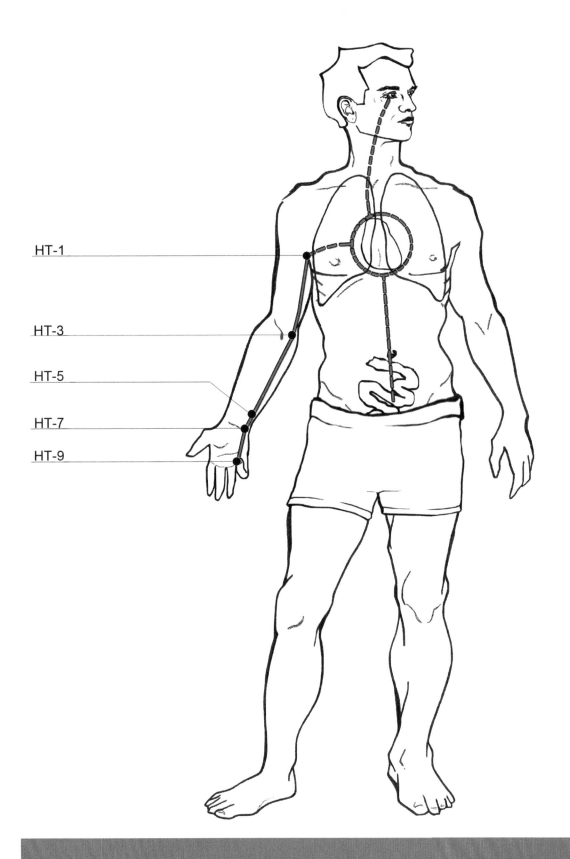

HT-1

HT-3

HT-5

HT-7

HT-9

HEART MERIDIAN | HAND SHAO YIN

Heart Meridian

Yin

Five Element perspective
Element: Fire (Cardinal Fire)
Yang partner: Small Intestine

Six Channel perspective
Heart channel of the hand Shao Yin
Partner: Kidney channel of the foot Shao Yin

Key points: HT-3, 5, 7

Beginning point: HT-1 in the center of the armpit

End point: HT-9 at the lateral nail bed of the pinky finger (when in anatomical position). This is the ring finger side of the pinky, which is more protected (Yin).

External pathway

This is a Yin meridian, so it will be on the inner arm surface. The Heart meridian is on the medial (pinky side) edge of the anterior surface of the forearm. It begins in the center of the armpit at HT-1 and runs along the medial border of the biceps muscle, to the medial edge of the elbow crease, along the forearm, and then crosses the palm of the hand to end at HT-9 located on the base of the fingernail of the pinky.

Internal pathway

The Heart meridian begins in the heart and then connects with the major blood vessels around the heart. The internal pathway branches, one branch connects to the small intestine, and another branch rises up through the throat to the eyes.

Think of the Heart meridian when:

There are mental, emotional, psychiatric conditions.
Dealing with anxiety, panic attacks.
There is insomnia.
There are cardiac conditions.

Approaching the Heart meridian

The Heart is the Emperor who is the ultimate commander of the entire Body–Mind. Common people are not allowed to chitchat with the Emperor, they are shuttled off to the bureaucrats (there is a hierarchy within the Organs just as in government). All this is to say that some traditional texts consider the Heart meridian off-limits to practitioners. Instead, use the Pericardium (as in talk to the assistant, not the Emperor).

The Heart is the Yin Organ of the most Yang Element—Cardinal Fire. The Heart, very importantly, is the house of the Shen. Shen is Spirit. The Shen resides in the sacred temple of the Heart. The Shen will scatter (resulting in emotional issues, and at the extreme, psychiatric conditions) if the Heart is not a calm, clear, nourishing home for it.

When we contact the Heart points it is best if our own Hearts are clear and calm for our Spirit's presence. From a state of reverence we reach out and make contact with the home of our client's Spirit.

Heart Points (HT-3, 5, 7)

HT-3: Shao Hai, "Lesser Sea"

Location: At the medial (pinky side) end of the anterior elbow crease.
Location tip: Bend the elbow in order to see the elbow crease. With the elbow bent it is easier to feel the large dip that marks this point on the anterior-medial edge of the crease.

Use:
To open the Heart meridian in order to support the whole upper arm
To relieve elbow pain and inflammation

HT-5: Tong Li, "Penetrating the Interior"

Location: 1 cun proximal from the wrist crease, on the ulnar edge of anterior forearm.
Location tip: Have client flex wrist slightly so you can feel the flexor carpi ulnaris tendon. HT-5 is on the thumb side of the tendon, 1 cun proximal to HT-7 (located at the wrist crease).

HT-5 is a Ma Dan Yang Heavenly Star Point.

Use:
To calm the Spirit

HT-7: Shen Men, "Spirit Gate"

Location: At the medial tip of the wrist crease, on the ulnar edge of anterior forearm.
Location tip: Have client flex wrist slightly so you can feel flexor carpi ulnaris tendon. HT-7 is on the thumb side of the tendon, located at the medial tip of the wrist crease.

HT-7 is the Yuan Source Point of the Heart meridian.

Use:
To calm the Spirit
To help with insomnia

Point combination:
HT-7 + REN-17 to calm the Spirit.

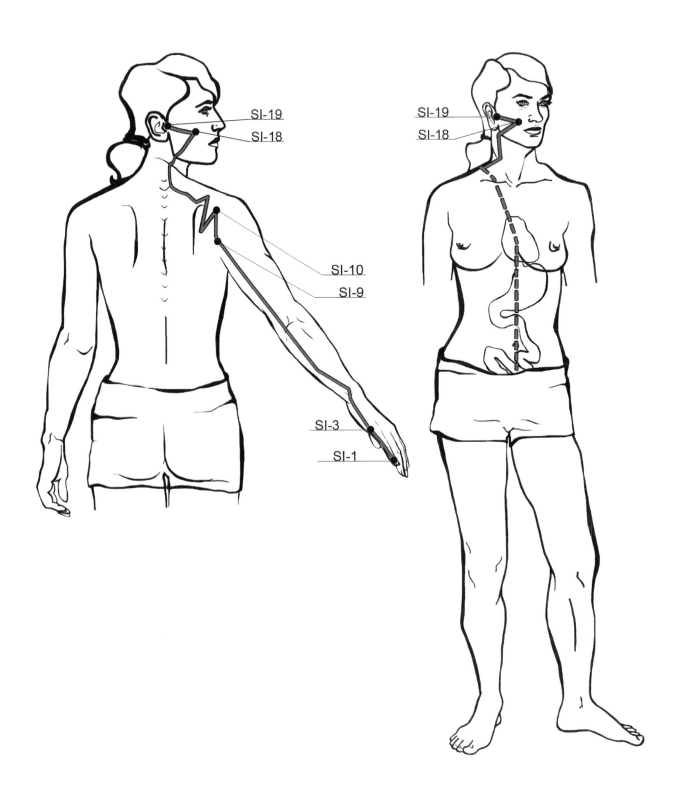

SI-19
SI-18
SI-10
SI-9
SI-3
SI-1
SI-19
SI-18

SMALL INTESTINE MERIDIAN | HAND TAI YANG

Small Intestine Meridian

Yang

Five Element perspective
Element: Fire (Cardinal)
Yin partner: Heart

Six Channel perspective
Small Intestine channel of the hand Tai Yang [19]
Partnered with Bladder channel of the foot Tai Yang

Key points: SI-3, 9, 10, 18, 19

Beginning point: SI-1 on the lateral nail bed of the pinky finger

End point: SI-19 at the tragus ("ear flap") of the ear

External pathway

Begins at SI-1, located on the pinky, on the nail bed opposite the HT-9. This is a Yang meridian, so it passes along the posterior aspect of the forearm on the medial edge, between the olecranon process of the ulna and medial epicondyle of the humerus, along the medial triceps to the posterior crease of the armpit, zigzags over the scapula and goes close to cervical vertebra C7, then up the lateral neck to the cheek, and ends just in front of the tragus of the ear at SI-19.

Internal pathway

An internal pathway branch passes to ST-12 and then goes down to the heart, the throat, and on down to the stomach, and then to the small intestine.

Think of the Small Intestine meridian when:

There is pain along the meridian pathway and especially posterior shoulder–scapula pain.
There is excess heat as in fevers, abscess, dryness or thirst, ulcers in the stomach or intestines, diverticulitis.

Approaching the Small Intestine meridian

This is the Yang meridian of the Fire Element, so it has everything to do with heat. Use the Small Intestine meridian to clear away excess heat. The Heart meridian is the Yin meridian of the Fire Element and is used to nourish the Heart and Blood, while the Small Intestine meridian is used to move out the excess heat.

Small Intestine Points (3, 9, 10, 18, 19)

SI-3: Hou Xi, "Back Stream"

Location: On the pinky edge of the hand just proximal to the fifth knuckle.
Location tip: Bend the pinky finger: The crease that is formed on the lateral edge of the hand marks the point.

SI-3 is a Master Point of the Du Vessel.[20] As the name implies, use SI-3:
To open the Du Vessel of the spine
To relieve pain in the neck, back

Point combination:
SI-3+ BL-62 for any issue of the vertebral column, neck pain.
(Master Point combination)

SI-9: Jian Zhen, "True Shoulder"

Location: Posterior shoulder, 1 cun superior to the axillary crease.
Location tip: Slide with gentle pressure up from the posterior axillary (armpit) crease and feel for a dip.

Use:
To open the shoulder joint, relieve shoulder pain
To open the Small Intestine meridian and relieve pain in the upper trapezius and neck

SI-10: Nao Shu, "Upper Arm Shu"

Location: Posterior shoulder, about 2 cun superior to the SI-9.
Location tip: Slide with gentle pressure up from SI-9 and feel for a dip. SI-10 is directly over the shoulder joint, SI-9 is below it.
Use:
To open the shoulder joint, relieve shoulder pain

To open the Small Intestine meridian and relieve pain in the upper trapezius and neck

SI-18: Quan Liao, "Cheek Bone Crevice"

Location: In a depression under the zygomatic bone, in line with the outer canthus of the eye.
Location tip: At the "edge" of the cheek bone, feel for the zygomatic bone in line with the outer canthus of the eye and apply pressure up from under the bone.

Use:
To relieve tooth pain, face and head pain

SI-19: Ting Gong, "Palace of Hearing"

Location: Just in front of the tragus of the ear.
Location tip: Have client open mouth: Feel for a dip between the tragus and the condyle of the mandible.

Use:
To open the ear, relieve pressure in the ear, tinnitus

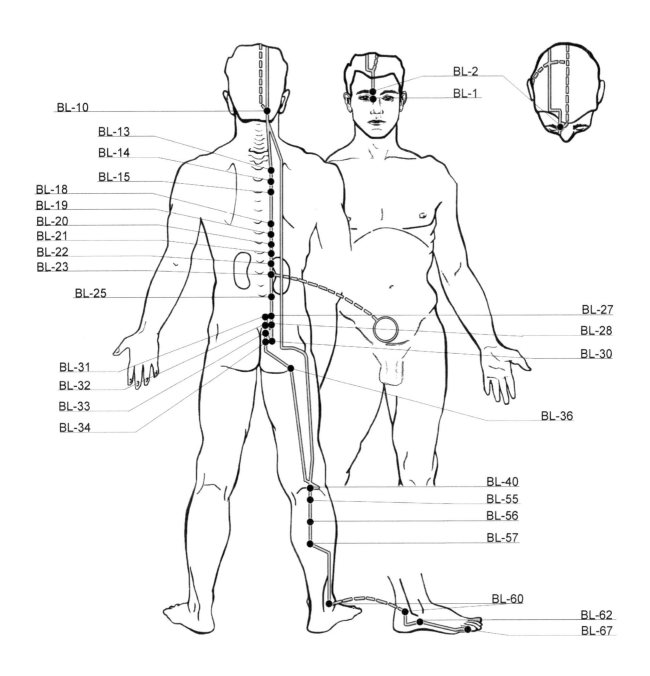

BLADDER MERIDIAN | FOOT TAI YANG

BL-2
BL-1
BL-10
BL-13
BL-14
BL-15
BL-18
BL-19
BL-20
BL-21
BL-22
BL-23
BL-25
BL-27
BL-28
BL-30
BL-31
BL-32
BL-33
BL-34
BL-36
BL-40
BL-55
BL-56
BL-57
BL-60
BL-62
BL-67

Bladder Meridian

Yang

Five Element perspective
Element: Water
Yin partner: Kidney

Six Channel perspective
Bladder channel of the foot Tai Yang
Partnered with Small Intestine channel of the hand Tai Yang

Key Points: BL-10, 13–28, 31–34, 36, 40, 55, 56, 57, 60, 62, 67

Beginning point: BL-1 at the inner canthus of the eye

Ending point: Lateral nail bed of the pinky toe

External pathway

This is a long one! It begins at BL-1, located at the inner corner of the eye, moves up over the head, then down the back to the pinky toe. The Bladder meridian has more points than any other meridian.

Once this meridian ascends the forehead, it goes over the head, down the back of the neck, and then divides into two pathways. The inner line is 1.5 cun lateral from the midline, the outer is 3 cun lateral. These two branches go down the entire back. The inner line traverses the sacral foramen, both lines cross the buttocks and then reunite at BL-40 (back of the knee). The inner line drops down to the center of the hamstrings and has the points on it; the outer line has no points on it (at the level of the hamstrings).

From BL-40 the BL meridian goes down the center of the gastrocnemius muscle. Then, at the junction of the Achilles tendon, it goes lateral and continues down the posterior–lateral edge of the lower leg, travels posterior to the lateral malleolus, along the lateral edge of the foot to end at BL-67 on the lateral nail bed of the pinky toe.

Internal pathway

The internal pathway breaks away from the inner back line in the lumbar area to connect with the kidneys and the bladder.

Think of the Bladder meridian when:

There is any pain along the meridian, especially back pain.
Dealing with conditions of the spine such as scoliosis and other curves.
To support the function of all the organs and overall health via the Shu points.

Approaching the Bladder meridian

This is the Yang meridian of the most Yin Element, Water. It covers the entire posterior aspect of the body, and is the location of the Shu points—an important set of points related to every organ in the body and discussed below.

Due to its location along the head, neck, and back, the Bladder meridian is susceptible to invasions of exterior pathogens. By keeping the meridian supplied with plenty of Qi, and keeping that Qi moving, we prevent these types of invasions.

Utilize this meridian to bring the overall Qi down, to ground the Mind and Spirit. Yang tends to rise, so working the BL meridian is great way to bring the Yang back down and keep it rooted in the body.

Bladder Points (10, 13–28, 31–34, 36, 40, 55, 56, 57, 60, 62, 67)

BL-10: Tian Zhu, "Celestial Pillar"

Location: Just below the occiput, a little more than 1 cun lateral to occipital notch.
Location tip: Find the occipital notch and move laterally over the attachment of the trapezius muscles, feeling for the point. (GB-20 is more lateral than BL-10.)

Use:
To relieve neck and head pain

BL-13–28: Back-Shu Points

Location: Level with the spinous process of the vertebrae given, 1.5 cun lateral to the spinous processes.
Location tip: These points are on the inner Bladder line located on the high point of the erector spinae group. Measure 1.5 cun lateral to the spine by locating the medial border of the scapula (3 cun lateral). Halfway between the spinous process and the medial border of the scapula is 1.5 cun.

Use:
These points "transport" Qi directly to the associated Organ. Use them to directly affect the physical organ. As a group, these points energize and support each of the Organs when stimulated.

POINT	PIN YIN	ENGLISH	VERTEBRAE
BL-13	Fei Shu	Lung Shu	T3
BL-14	Jue Yin Shu	Pericardium Shu	T4
BL-15	Xin Shu	Heart Shu	T5
BL-18	Gan Shu	Liver Shu	T9
BL-19	Dan Shu	Gallbladder Shu	T10
BL-20	Pi Shu	Spleen Shu	T11
BL-21	Wei Shu	Stomach Shu	T12
BL-22	San Jiao Shu	San Jiao Shu	L1
BL-23	Shen Shu	Kidney Shu	L2
BL-25	Da Chang Shu	Large Intestine Shu	L4
BL-27	Xiao Chang Shu	Small Intestine Shu	S1
BL-28	Pang Guan Shu	Bladder Shu	S2

BL-31: Shang Liao, "Upper Crevice"

Location: On the sacrum in the first sacral foramen.
Location tip: The foramen are quite medial. Locate the center line of the sacrum and inch laterally and feel for the dip of the foramen. The dip is the point.

Use:*
To open the back BL meridian, bring the Qi down
To relieve pain in the sacral-lumbar area
To support the functions of the bladder, uterus, rectum
*BL-31 is contra-indicated in pregnancy

BL-32: Ci Liao, "Second Crevice"

Location: On the sacrum in the second sacral foramen
Location tip: Same as BL-31.

Of the four sacral points, BL-32 is the most important, the "Big Deal" point. Use it:
To open the back BL meridian, bring the Qi down
To relieve pain in the sacral-lumbar area
To support the functions of the bladder, uterus, rectum
*BL-32 is contra-indicated in pregnancy

BL-33: Zhong Liao, "Middle Crevice"

Location: On the sacrum in the third sacral foramen.
Location tip: Same as BL-31.

Use:*
To open the back BL meridian, bring the Qi down
To relieve pain in the sacral-lumbar area
To support the functions of the bladder, uterus, rectum
*BL-33 is contra-indicated in pregnancy

BL-34: Xia Liao, "Lower Crevice"

Location: On the sacrum in the fourth sacral foramen
Location tip: Same as BL-31.

Use:
To open the back BL meridian, bring the Qi down
To relieve pain in the sacral-lumbar area
To support the functions of the bladder, uterus, rectum
*BL-34 is contra-indicated in pregnancy

BL-36: Cheng Fu, "Hold and Support"

Location: Just below the ischial tuberosity.
Location tip: Located directly on the upper attachments of the hamstrings.

Use:
To open the back BL meridian, bring the Qi down
To relieve pain in the sacral-lumbar area
To support the hamstrings

BL-40: Wei Zhong, "Middle of the Crook"

Location: Center of the posterior knee.
Location tip: Use the thumb and finger of one hand to contact the sides of the knee, now locate the point in the center of your contact.

BL-40 is:
1) A Ma Dan Yang Heavenly Star Point
2) Command Point of the back

Use:
To relieve all types of back pain, especially the lower back
For local knee pain

BL 55: He Yang, "Confluence of Yang"

Location: Center of the gastrocnemius (calf muscle) 2 cun distal toward the foot) from BL-40.
Location tip: Locate BL-40 in the center of the posterior (back) knee, slide directly down 2 cun in the midline of the gastrocnemius. BL-55 is at the top of the gastrocnemius, BL-56 is in the center, BL-57 is at the lower (distal) end of the gastrocnemius.

Use:
To relieve low back pain

Point combination:
BL-55, 56, 57 + BL-23 to relieve low back pain

BL-56: Cheng Jin, "Support the Sinews"

Location: In the center of the gastrocnemius, 5 cun inferior to BL-40, on the midline of the gastrocnemius.
Location tip: BL-55 is at the top of the gastrocnemius, BL-56 is in the center, BL-57 is at the lower (distal) end of the gastrocnemius.

Use:
To relieve local calf pain
To open the BL meridian above the point, help clear the head, neck, and back

Point combination:
BL-55, 56, 57 + BL-23 to relieve low back pain

BL-57: Cheng Shan, "Support the Mountain"

Location: On the midline of the gastrocnemius where the Achilles tendon meets the lower heads of the gastrocnemius.
Location tip: BL-55 is at the top of the gastrocnemius, BL-56 is in the center, BL-57 is at the lower (distal) end of the gastrocnemius.

BL-57 is a Ma Dan Yang Heavenly Star Point.

Use:
To relieve local calf pain
To open the BL meridian above the point, help clear the head, neck, and back
To relieve hemorrhoids

Point combination:
BL-55, 56, 57 + BL-23 to relieve low back pain

BL-60: Kun Lun, "Kunlun Mountains"

Location: Opposite Kidney meridian point KD-3 on the lateral aspect of the Achilles tendon, posterior to the lateral malleolus.
Location tip: Measure halfway between the high point of the lateral malleolus (outer ankle bone) and the Achilles tendon.

BL-60 is a Ma Dan Yang Heavenly Star Point.

Use:*
To open the BL meridian above the point, help clear the head, neck, and back
To bring the Qi down
*Contra-indicated in pregnancy

BL-62: Shen Mai, "Extending Vessel"

Location: Half a cun below the lateral malleolus.
Location tip: Slide down from the lateral malleolus and feel for the dip.

Use:
This is the Master Point of the Yang Qiao Vessel. [21]
It opens the whole meridian and so relieves stagnation from head to toe.
Use it to calm the Spirit.

Point combination:

BL-62 + SI-3 for back pain and neck pain, disc issues, spinal cord issues.

BL-67: Zhi Yin, "Reaching Yin"

Location: Lateral aspect of the nail bed of the little toe.

Use:*
To open the BL meridian above the point, help clear the head, neck, and back
*In pregnancy this point turns the fetus in the case of a breach position and encourages labor. Therefore this point is contraindicated during pregnancy and used only when the Mother is full term and ready to give birth.

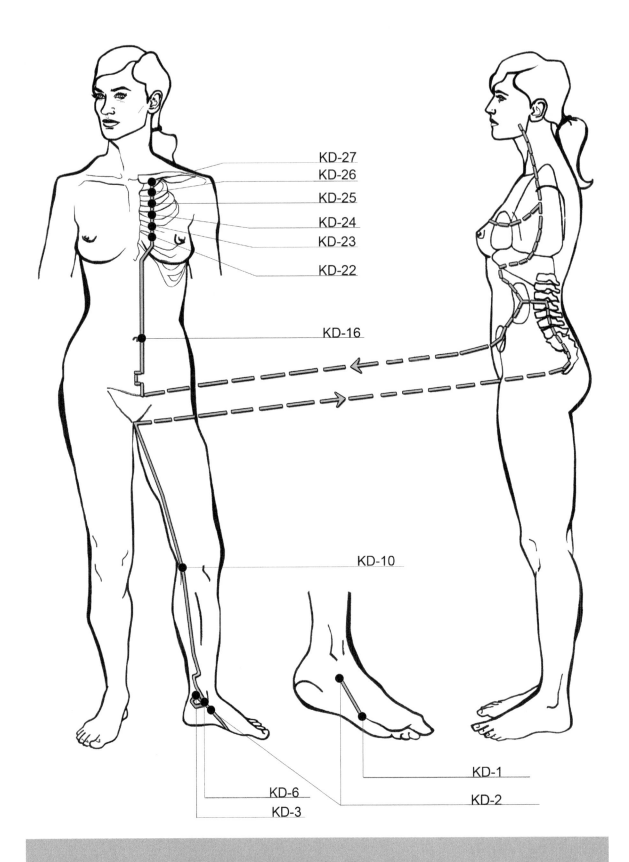

KD-27
KD-26
KD-25
KD-24
KD-23
KD-22

KD-16

KD-10

KD-1
KD-2

KD-6
KD-3

KIDNEY MERIDIAN | FOOT SHAO YIN

Kidney Meridian

Yin

Five Element perspective
Element: Water
Yang partner: Bladder

Six Channel perspective
Kidney channel of the foot Shao Yang [22]
Partner: Heart channel of the hand Shao Yang

Key points: KD-1, 2, 3, 6, 10, 22–27

Beginning point: KD-1 on the sole of the foot one-third the distance toward the heel from the toes, between the second and third metatarsals

End point: KD-27, just below the clavicle at the lateral edge of the manubrium (top of the breast bone)

External pathway

Kidney 1 is located on the bottom of the foot, the lowest place in the body, the most Yin place. From the bottom of the foot, the Kidney meridian comes across midway on the medial arch of the foot to the heel, circles around the medial heel, and then proceeds up the posterior edge of the medial leg and thigh. At the inguinal area, it dives internally and pops out again in the pubic region to travel up the abdomen (.5 cun lateral to the navel). At the lower ribs, the meridian moves laterally and continues up lateral to the sternum and ends just lateral to the manubrium and inferior to the medial clavicle.

Internal pathway

The Kidneys are the containers of our Life Force, so it makes sense that this meridian would make more connections than other meridians do—and it does. There are many branches off the main meridian that run internally, and branches from internal pathways that go even further. Here is the summary:

From the thigh, the internal pathway continues up and enters the spinal column from the coccyx, goes up to the top of the column, and then comes back down again. A branch enters the kidneys, bladder, and uterus. Another branch goes to the liver, diaphragm, lungs, and heart.

Think of the Kidney meridian when:

There are any bone conditions.
There are growth and development issues.
There are issues with aging, longevity, premature aging, general constitution.
There are issues with fertility.
There are issues with sexual organs and their functions.
There are difficult symptoms around menopause.
There are problems with the central nervous system—brain and spinal cord—condition.

Approaching the Kidney meridian

The Life Force is held within the Kidneys. When you contact the Kidney meridian, you are contacting the eternal, sacred, mysterious Life Force that expresses itself with this particular person. Allow yourself to be in reverence, stillness, and guided by the Mysterious as you sink into this most Yin of all meridians.

If we are to preserve our Life Force, we must attend to our Kidneys. The Kidney meridian is the Yin meridian of the most Yin Element, Water. The Kidneys store our Jing, the pre-Heaven Essence we received at conception.

If we are exhausting ourselves with a busy lifestyle that does not include restoring our post-Heaven Qi well, we tap into our Jing to keep going. This can be thought of as our reserves, our "bounce-back." Longevity is tied to the Kidneys for this reason. We run out of life when we run out of Jing.

Jing is to be protected, consolidated, not wasted or leaked. Nourish, warm, and protect the Kidneys and the Kidney meridian.

Kidney points (1, 2, 3, 6, 10, 22–27)

KD-1: Yong Quan, "Bubbling Spring"

Location: On the sole of the foot between the second and third metatarsals, one-third of the distance from the base of the second toe to the heel.
Location tip: Slide toward the heel from between the second and third toe feeling for a dip.

This is the lowest point on the body.

Use:
To bring energy down from the head
To support connection to the Earth

KD-2: Ran Gu, "Blazing Valley"

Location: On the arch of the foot, just posterior to the anterior tibialis tendon.
Location tip: Have the client invert and dorsiflex the foot and you will see the tibialis anterior tendon clearly. Locate a dip just posterior to the tendon as it comes to the arch. (SP-4 is distal to this tendon, KD-2 is proximal to it.)

Use:
To relieve hot flashes

KD-3: Tai Xi, "Supreme Stream"

Location: On the medial aspect of the ankle, halfway between the medial malleolus and the Achilles tendon.
Location tip: Look and feel for the depression halfway between the medial malleolus and the Achilles tendon.

KD-3 is the Yuan Source Point of the Kidney meridian and an extremely important point, as the Kidneys hold the Life Force.

Use:
To nourish the Kidneys, consolidate Kidney Qi
As a key point to nourish Yin in the entire body-mind

Point combination:
KD-3 + BL-60 to bring the Qi down from the head.

KD-6: Zhao Hai, "Shining Sea"

Location: 1 cun inferior to the high point of the medial malleolus.
Location tip: Gently slide inferiorly (down toward the sole of foot) from the high point of the medial malleolus and feel for the groove between the ligaments there.

This the Master Point of the Yin Qiao. [23]

Use:
To nourish Kidney Yin
To help relieve hot flashes, night sweats

Point combination:
KD-6 + LU-7 stimulates the Yin of the entire body.

KD-10: Yin Gu, "Yin Valley"

Location: Medial knee, at the popliteal crease between the hamstring tendons semitendinosus and semimembranosus.
Location tip: Feel behind the medial knee for the two hamstring tendons. The point is located level with the knee crease between these tendons.

Use:
For local knee pain
To support the Kidneys

KD-22–27

KD-22: Bu Lang, "Walking Corridor
KD-23: Shen Feng, "Spirit Seal"
KD-24: Ling Xu, "Spirit Ruins"
KD-25: Shen Cang, "Spirit Storehouse"
KD-26: Yu Zhong, "Comfortable Chest"
KD-27: Shu Fu, "Shu Mansion"

Location: 2 cun lateral to the midline. KD-22 is in the fifth intercostal space. Each progressive point is one space superior to end at KD-27, which is located at the corner of the manubrium and medial clavicle.
Location tip: Slide fingers into the intercostal spaces just lateral to the sternum. The points are located 2 cun lateral to the midline of the sternum between the ribs.

Use:
To open the breath
To support the connection and communication of Fire (Heart) and Water (Kidney)

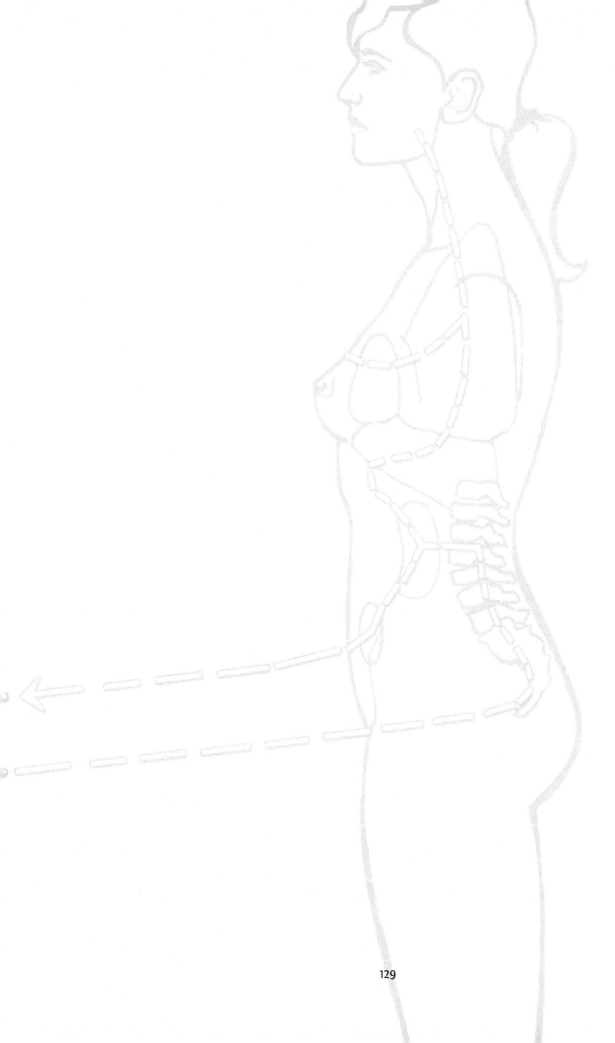

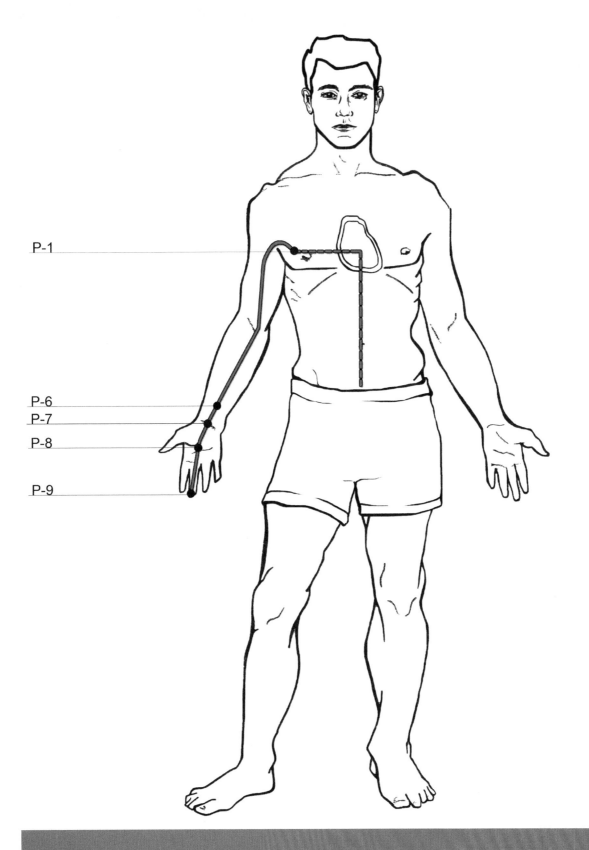

P-1

P-6
P-7

P-8

P-9

PERICARDIUM MERIDIAN | HAND JUE YIN

Pericardium Meridian

Yin

Five Element perspective
Element: Fire (supplemental)
Yang partner: San Jiao

Six Channel perspective
Pericardium channel of the hand Jue Yin
Partner: Liver channel of the foot Jue Yin

Key points: P-6, 7, 8

Beginning point: P-1 located 1 cun lateral to the nipple

End point: P-9 at the tip of the middle finger

External pathway

Begins at P-1, just lateral to the nipple and travels along the center of the anterior surface of the upper arm and forearm, crosses the palm, and ends at P-9, located on the tip of the third finger.

Internal pathway

Begins in the center chest, goes to the pericardium and follows the aorta down through the diaphragm and connects with the San Jiao. The San Jiao, or three warmers, is/are purely energetic, there is no physical form associated with the San Jiao.

Think of the Pericardium meridian when:

There are cardiac issues.
There are emotional issues similar to those associated with the Heart, as this is the meridian often used to treat the Heart (Remember: Talk to the assistant, not the Emperor).
Dealing with hormonal balance/imbalance.

Approaching the Pericardium meridian

This is a Yin meridian, so bring nourishment, quiet, and calm rather than motion and vigor. Use the Pericardium to benefit the Heart. This meridian also referred to as the "Heart Protector" so consider approaching the Pericardium with care—especially when you feel the client shows a sense of vulnerability and/or protectiveness.

Pericardium points (P-6, 7, 8)

P-6: Nei Guan, "Inner Gate"

Location: Anterior forearm, 2 cun proximal from the wrist crease on the center line.
Location tip: With the wrist slightly flexed, follow the palmaris tendon proximally 2 cun proximally (toward the elbow). The point is on the ulnar side of the palmaris tendon.

P-6 is
1) Command Point of the chest
2) Master Point of the Yin Wei

Use:
To calm the Spirit
To open the chest
To soothe nausea

Point combinations:
P-6 + SP-4 to calm the interior, bring the attention inward, and help the client rest.
P-6 + REN-17 disperses Qi in the chest, calms the heart, soothes stressed heart/mind.

P-7: Da Ling, "Great Mound"

Location: In the center of the anterior wrist crease.
Location tip: Slightly flex the wrist to show the wrist crease plainly. P-7 is in the center of the crease.
P-7 is the Yuan Source Point for the Pericardium meridian.

Use:
To nourish the Heart
To calm the Spirit

P-8: Lao Gong, "Palace of Toil"

Location: On the palm of the hand, between the second and third metacarpal bones, proximal to the knuckles.
Location tip: Make a gentle fist. Where the middle finger contacts the palm is the location of the point.

This is an important point for hands-on practitioners as a place of offering our Qi to another person.

Use:
Use it to calm the Spirit.

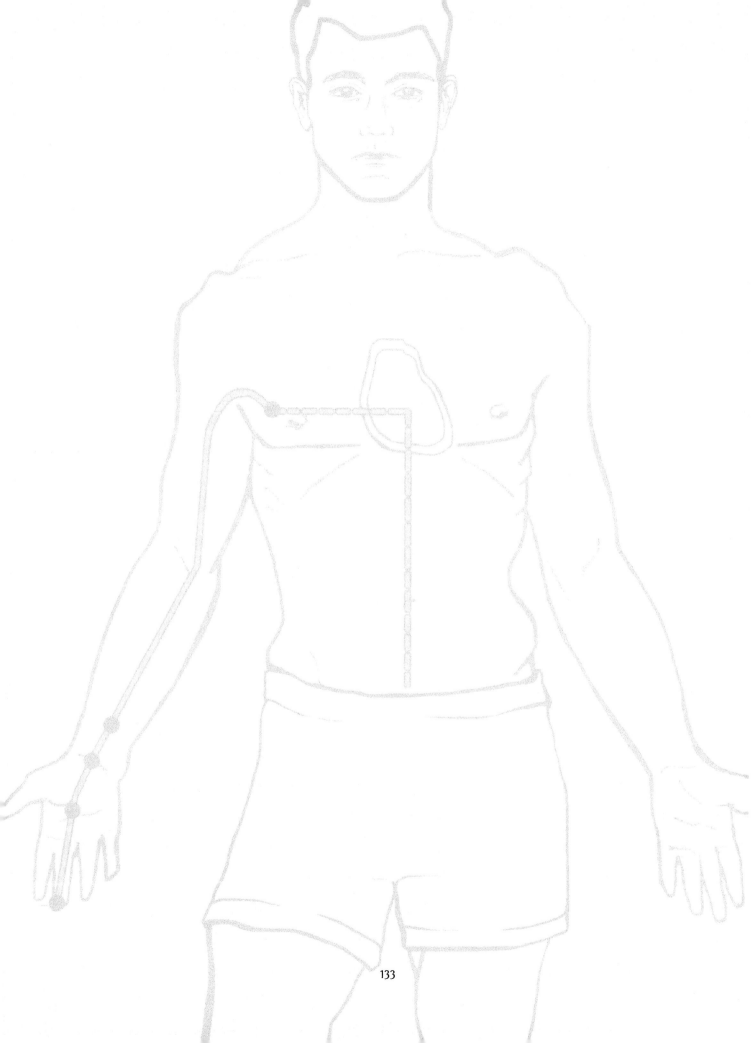

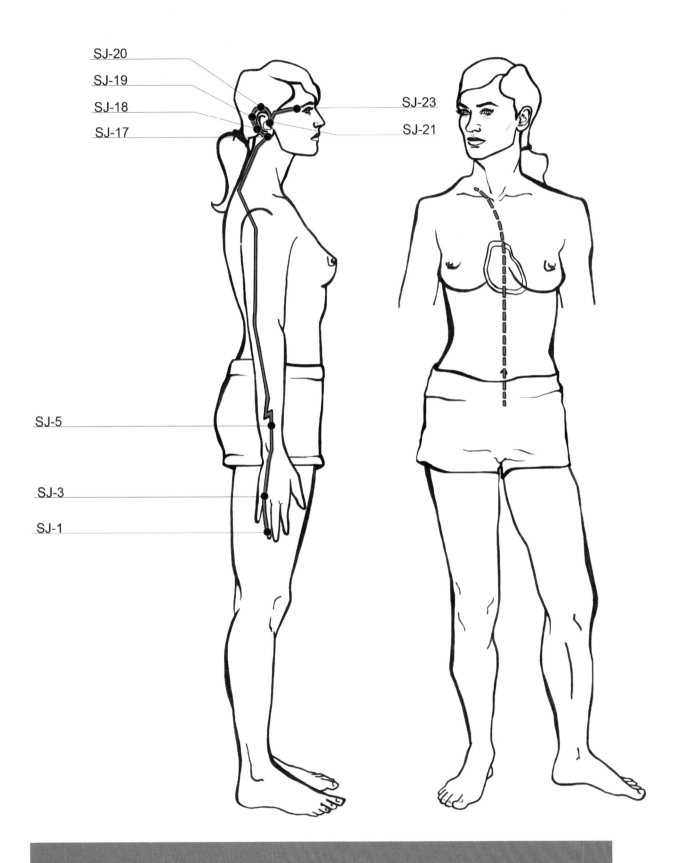

SJ-20
SJ-19
SJ-18
SJ-17
SJ-23
SJ-21
SJ-5
SJ-3
SJ-1

SAN JAIO MERIDIAN | HAND SHAO YANG

San Jiao Meridian

Yang

Five Element perspective
Fire (Supplemental)
Yin partner: Pericardium

Six Channel perspective
San Jiao channel of the hand Shao Yang
Partnered: Gallbladder channel of the foot Shao Yang

Key points: SJ-3, 5, 21

Beginning point: SJ-1 on the lateral nail bed of the fourth finger

End point: SJ-23 at the lateral tip of the eyebrow

External pathway

Begins at SJ-1 located on the lateral nail bed of the ring finger, runs along the center of the posterior aspect of the forearm, between the olecranon of the ulna and the lateral epicondyle of the humerus, up the center of the triceps, across the posterior upper trapezius, up the lateral neck to the soft spot behind the ear lobe, goes around the posterior ear to just in front of the tragus, then ends at the lateral tip of the eyebrow, at SJ-23.

Internal pathway

From the posterior upper trapezius, the internal branch breaks away and goes to ST-12. From ST-12 it passes down to REN-17, onward to the pericardium, continues through the diaphragm and connects the three warmers. There is no actual triple warm (San Jiao) physical organ; these are purely energetic.

Think of the San Jiao meridian when:

There are excess heat issues such as fever, red-dry conditions, ulcers, abscess, high blood pressure, hot temper, anxiety, hyperactivity.
There is a one-sided headache.
There is an ear infection or ear pain.
There is pain anywhere along the external pathway.

Approaching the San Jiao meridian

This is a Yang meridian, so use vigor and movement to get the Qi moving! The San Jiao meridian has a relationship with the Gallbladder meridian in Six Channel theory, so include this meridian when you need to resolve one-sided complaints.

San Jiao points (SJ-3, 5, 21)

SJ-3: Zhong Zhu, "Central Islet"

Location: On the dorsum of the hand, just proximal to the fourth and fifth knuckles.
Location tip: Slide with gentle pressure proximally (toward the wrist) from between the fourth and fifth knuckles, feeling for the dip that marks the point.

This is an influential point for the ear.

Use:
For acute ear pain
For ear infection
To relieve air pressure blocks while flying

SJ-5: Wai Guan, "Outer Gate"

Location: 2 cun proximal to posterior wrist crease in the center of forearm.
Location tip: Slide gently 2 cun proximally from the center of posterior wrist crease feeling for the dip.

Master Point of the Yang Wei Vessel. [24]

Use:
To clear heat from the body
To open the San Jiao meridian to relieve stagnation anywhere in the meridian
To relieve ear pain, inflammation, heat

Point combination:
SJ-5 + GB-41 to relieve neck pain and one sided tension patterns.

SJ-21: Er Men, "Ear Gate"

Location: Just in front of the tragus.
Location tip: Apply gentle pressure just anterior to the tragus to feel for a dip between the tragus and the condyle of the mandible. There are three points in this groove: SJ-21 is toward the top, SI-19 is in the middle, and GB-2 is at the lower end.

Use:
To relieve ear issues such as infection, pain, stuffiness
To open the jaw and relieve tension

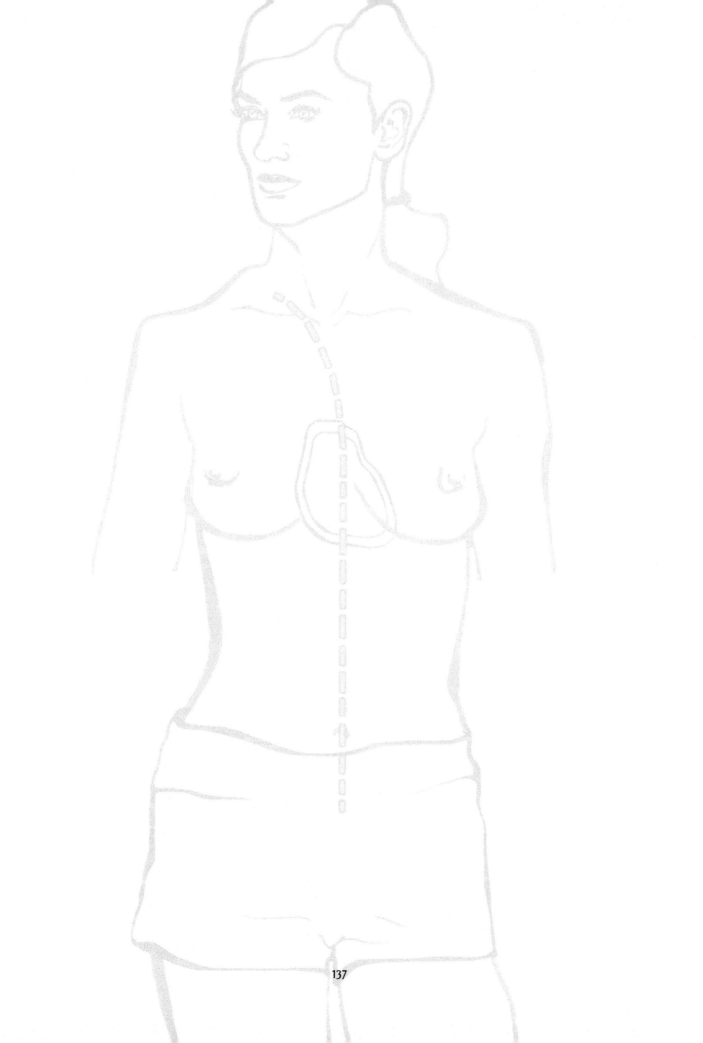

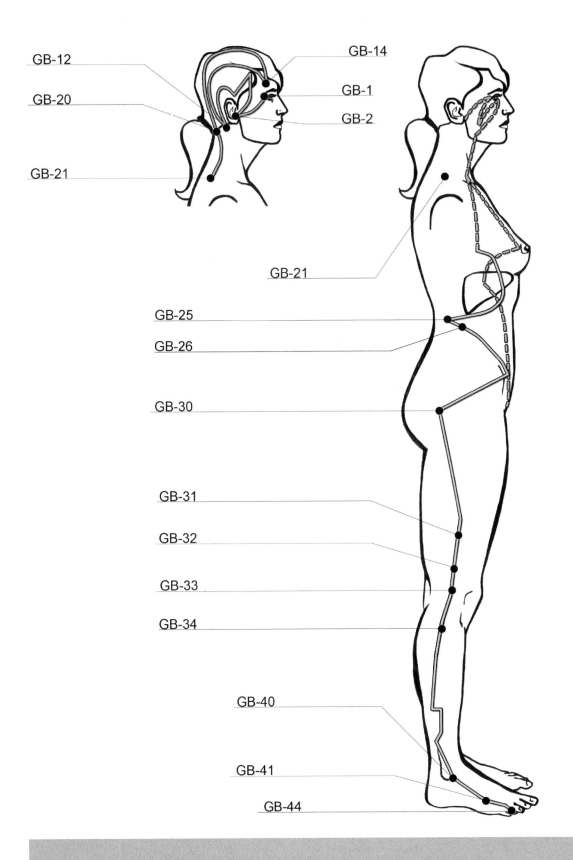

GB-12
GB-20
GB-21
GB-14
GB-1
GB-2
GB-21
GB-25
GB-26
GB-30
GB-31
GB-32
GB-33
GB-34
GB-40
GB-41
GB-44

GALLBLADDER MERIDIAN | FOOT SHAO YANG

Gallbladder Meridian

Yang

Five Element perspective
Element: Wood
Yin partner: Liver

Six Channel perspective
Gallbladder channel of the foot Shao Yang
Partner: San Jiao of the hand Shao Yang

Key points: GB-1, 2, 12, 14, 20, 21, 25, 26, 30–34, 40, 41

Beginning point: GB-1 at the outer canthus of the eye

End point: GB-44 at the lateral nail bed of the fourth toe

External pathway

From GB-1 at the lateral canthus of the eye, this meridian travels to the tragus of the ear, then zigzags on the side of the head, to the occipital bone, to the upper trapezius where it goes inside to pop out again on the lateral rib cage between the fifth and sixth ribs, then zigs and zags along the side of the trunk, goes to the lateral hip, down the iliotibial tract, past the side of the knee, the head of the fibula, down the center of the lateral leg, across the lateral malleolus, across the top of the foot to end at the lateral nail bed of the fourth toe.

Internal pathway

From the point GB-21 on the upper trapezius, an internal branch goes anterior to ST-12 where it descends through the diaphragm, connects to the liver and gallbladder, then circles around the interior rib cage, and goes down to the inguinal area to connect with the point ST-30.

Think of the Gallbladder meridian when:

There are one-sided conditions.
There are one-sided headaches.
The client has a short temper, is stressed, revved up, ready to explode, wound up, tense, angry, has tight tendons.
There is sciatica.

Hip pain.

Jaw pain and tension.

Approaching the Gallbladder meridian:

This is the Yang meridian of the Wood Element, of Spring. Qi stagnation is often an issue, and the Gallbladder meridian is a site of lots of Qi stagnation—so let's get it moving! Vigorous movements really help the Gallbladder open up. Be aware that your client may experience some zingy pain (go easy) as things get going, and then may drop into a state of deep relaxation and stillness as the Qi moves and resettles.

Gallbladder points (GB-1, 2, 12, 14, 20, 21, 25, 26, 30–34, 40, 41)

GB 1: Tong Zi Liao, "Pupil Crevice"

Location: At the lateral corner (canthus) of the eye.

Location tip: Move slowly here in order to support the client feeling safe as you apply pressure so close to the eye.

Use:

To relieve any eye issues

GB-2: Ting Hui, "Meeting of Hearing"

Location: Just in front of the tragus.

Location tip: Apply gentle pressure just anterior to the tragus to feel for dip between the tragus and the condyle of the mandible. There are three points in this groove: SJ-21 is toward the top, SI-19 is in the middle, and GB-2 is at the lower end.

Use:

To relieve ear issues, infection, pain, stuffiness

To open the jaw and relieve tension

GB-12: Wan Gu, "Mastoid Process"

Location: Just posterior to the mastoid process.

Location tip: Locate the mastoid process then roll your finger posterior to it, feeling for a dip.

Use:

To relieve headaches

GB-14: Yang Bai, "Yang White"

Location: On the forehead, 1 cun directly superior to the eyebrow, in line with the pupil.
Location tip: As the client looks forward, note the location of the pupil and then find the dip in the forehead directly above the pupil on the forehead and 1 cun above the eyebrow.

Use:
To relieve headaches
To relieve tension in the forehead
To relieve eye strain, pain

GB-20: Feng Chi, "Wind Pool"

Location: Just below the occiput bone halfway between GB-12 and DU-16 (occipital notch).
Location tip: Feel for the muscle attachments of the erector spinae onto the occiput, move a little lateral and feel for the point. Your client will be very helpful telling you when you are on the point as this is often sore.

Of all of the head GB points, GB-20 is the most powerful for relieving headaches.

Use:
To relieve headaches
To relieve dizziness
To relieve neck pain

GB-21: Jian Jing, "Shoulder Well"

Location: On the upper trapezius halfway between the spinous process of C7 and the acromion process.
Location tip: This is the classic "sore spot" in the upper trapezius. Squeeze the upper trapezius feeling for the "knot" about half way between the side of the neck and the edge of the shoulder. Apply pressure gently as this is often very tender.

Working this point strongly moves Qi down.

Use:*
To open the shoulders, relieve pain and tension in the neck and shoulders
To relieve headaches
*Contraindicated in pregnancy

GB-25: Jing Men, "Capital Gate"

Location: Just below the tip of the twelfth rib

Location tip: Gently locate the twelfth rib and slowly sink pressure into the tissue at the end of the rib. This is often very tender, so move slowly.

Use:
To free the movement of the ribs in breathing
To open Qi flow through the side of the body

GB-26: Dai Mai, "Belt Vessel"

Location: About 1 cun inferior to the end of the eleventh rib.
Location tip: Located on the lateral abdomen, level with the navel and inferior to the free end of the eleventh rib.

Use:
To relieve pain or spasm of the ascending colon

GB-30: Huan Tiao, "Jumping Circle"

Location: Posterior-lateral hip, one-third the distance from the greater trochanter to the sacral-coccyx joint.
Location tip: With the client prone, apply gentle and gradual pressure as this is often very tender. Feel for the greater trochanter and the sacral-coccyx joint, then find the mark one-third of the distance from the great trochanter. Your client will tell you when you are on the point!

GB-30 is a Ma Dan Yang Heavenly Star Point.

Use:
To relieve hip pain
To relieve sciatic pain, especially when due to a tight piriformis muscle
To relieve one-sided headaches, as it clears the whole meridian

GB-31: Feng Shi, "Wind Market"

Location: On the lateral thigh where the middle finger naturally falls when standing with the arms at the side.
Location tip: Use your client's hand to guide you to the location on the lateral thigh. With arms at sides, where their middle finger contacts their thigh will be the point.
Use:
To relieve hip pain
To open the GB meridian

To relieve pain and tension in the iliotibial tract
To relieve knee pain

GB-32, Zhong Du, "Middle Ditch"

Location: 2 cun distal to GB-31.
Location tip: Slide toward the knee from GB-31 two inches (cun) and feel for a dip. Your client will also tell you when they feel a painful spot. "Ouch" means that you have located the point.

Use:
To relieve pain and tension in the iliotibial tract
To relieve knee pain

GB-33: Xi Yang Guan, "Knee Yang Gate"

Location: Lateral knee, just superior to the lateral condyle of femur and anterior to biceps femoris tendon.
Location tip: Slide toward the knee from GB-32 a few inches and feel for a dip just above the knee on the lateral aspect of the thigh. Your client will also tell you when they feel a painful spot. Again, "ouch" means that you have located the point.

Use:
For knee pain
To open the GB meridian

GB-34: Yang Ling Quan, "Yang Mound Spring"

Location: 1 cun anterior and inferior to the head of the fibula.
Location tip: Slide down 1 cun and then 1 cun anterior off of the head of the fibula and feel for the point.

GB-34 is:
1) A Ma Dan Yang Heavenly Star Point
2) The Influential Point for the sinews.

Use:
To move the Qi in the GB meridian
To relieve pain at the knee
To relieve one-sided issues
To strengthen the tendons
To heal tendon injuries anywhere in the body

GB-40: Qiu Xu, "Mound of Ruins"

Location: Lateral and inferior to the high point of the lateral malleolus.
Location tip: Have client invert foot. Look for the large depression that appears inferior to the lateral malleolus—that is the point.

Use:
To relieve ankle and lower leg pain
To open the GB meridian and help get the Qi moving

GB-41: Zu Lin Qi, "Foot Governor of Tears"

Location: On the dorsal surface of the foot, in the tiny depression lateral to the pinky fork of the extensor digitorum longus tendon.
Location tip: Have client extend toes (draw toes toward the nose) so you can locate the tendon. Then slide pressure proximally (toward the ankle) from between the fourth and fifth toes over the tendon. Immediately on the lateral aspect of the tendon, feel for the point.

Use:
GB-41 is the Master Point of the Dai Mai Vessel.[25] Use it
To relieve local pain and neck pain

Point combination:
GB-41 + SJ-5 for neck pain.

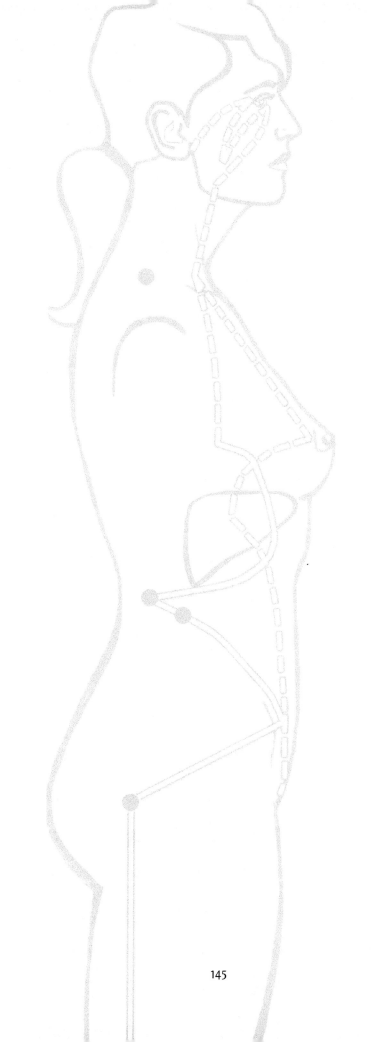

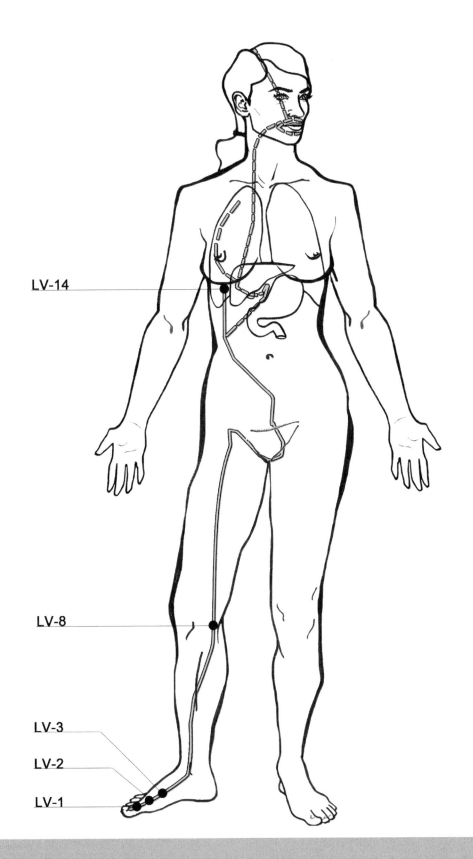

LV-14

LV-8

LV-3

LV-2

LV-1

LIVER MERIDIAN | FOOT JUE YIN

Liver Meridian

Yin

Five Element perspective
Element: Wood
Yang partner: Gallbladder

Six Channel perspective
Liver channel of the foot Jue Yin
Partner: Pericardium channel of hand Jue Yin

Key points: LV-2, 3, 8

Beginning point: LV-1 on the lateral aspect of the big toe nail

End point: LV-14 on the ribs, on mammillary line (just below the nipple or 4 cun lateral to the midsagittal line of the abdomen) in the sixth intercostal space

External pathway

From LV-1 on the lateral nail bed of the big toe the external pathway of the Liver meridian travels up the center of the medial aspect of the lower leg and thigh, crosses the anterior hip joint, circles the external reproductive organs, moves up the lateral aspect of the abdomen and ends at LV-14 located 6 cun lateral to the midline at the sixth intercostal space (between the sixth and seventh ribs).

Internal pathway

From the upper thigh, the internal pathway dives into the pelvis and wraps the internal reproductive organs, goes up the center of the inner abdomen to the stomach, the gallbladder and the liver. Another inner pathway continues up to the lungs, the throat, the eyes, and then to the top of the head to DU-20.

Think of the Liver meridian when:

Wood Element issues of anger, frustration, stress, tension are all signs of Qi stagnation in the body and mind. The Liver is responsible for the smooth flow of Qi: Like a gentle fan that keeps the air moving in room, the Liver keeps the Qi flowing. When Qi stagnates there are signs of physical pain and emotional stagnation.

Think of the Liver meridian for:
Menstrual cramps and irregularities.
Painful conditions of the sexual organs.
Headaches at the top of the head.
"Stressed out" mind-set.

Approaching the Liver meridian

Although this is a Yin meridian, it is the Yin meridian of the Wood, Spring, Element. In order to get the Qi flowing, it is often necessary to work some of the Liver points more vigorously than we generally would do on Yin meridians. This can be a very sensitive meridian, so even though we are bringing vigor, we do it gently and gradually.

Liver points (LV-2, 3, 8)

LV-2: Xing Jian, "Moving Between"

Location: On the dorsum (top) of the foot, in the web between the first and second toes, 0.5 cun proximal the base of the toes.
Location tip: Move just half an inch toward the ankle from the web between the big toe and second toes. Gently squeeze this point and ask the client to feel for an "ouch."

Use:
This point clears heat especially related to Liver/Wood issues such as
High blood pressure
Sudden headache or migraine
Dry itchy eyes
Hot temper
Hot flashes
Red face
Toxins in the blood such as medications, drugs, or alcohol.
Use it to clear heat.

LV-3: Tai Chong, "Great Rushing"

Location: On the dorsum of the foot, in a depression in the web between the first and second toes proximal to the big toe joint.
Location tip: Slide gentle pressure proximally from LV-2 and feel for the depression. This point is often very tender, so apply pressure gently.

LV-3 is:

1) Yuan Source Point of the Liver meridian

2) A Ma Dan Yang Heavenly Star Point

Use:

To soothe and calm the Liver

To move the Liver Qi to break up stagnation anywhere in the meridians

To relieve "stressed" mind-set

Point combination:

LV-3 + LI-4 are known as "the four gates" and are used in combination to open and move the Qi throughout the meridian system.

LV-8: Qu Quan, "Spring at the Crook"

Location: Medial knee, just superior to the medial knee crease.

Location tip: This point is very close to KD-10. KD-10 is more posterior, LV-8 is more medial. Apply gentle pressure at the end of the medial knee crease.

Use:

The Liver meridian wraps around the genitals and supports Liver Blood—which is especially helpful for women with heavy menstruation. Use LV-8

To relieve conditions affecting the genitals

To nourish the Blood generally and support Liver Blood in particular

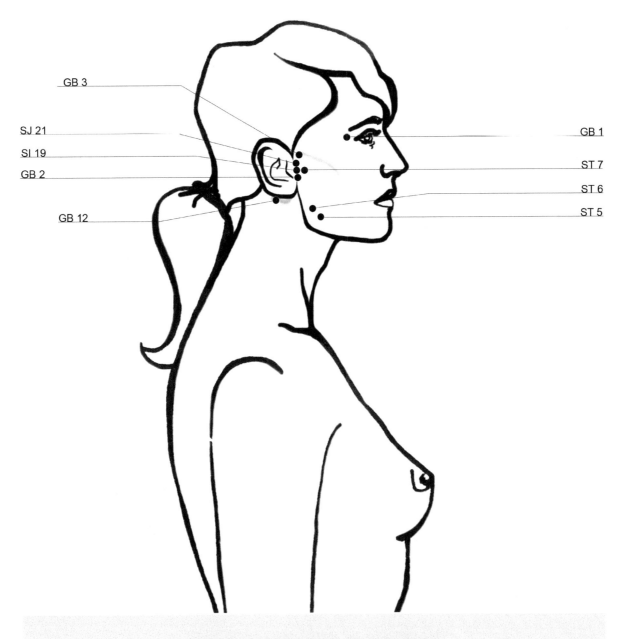

GB 3

SJ 21

SI 19

GB 2

GB 12

GB 1

ST 7

ST 6

ST 5

POINTS ON THE SIDE OF THE FACE

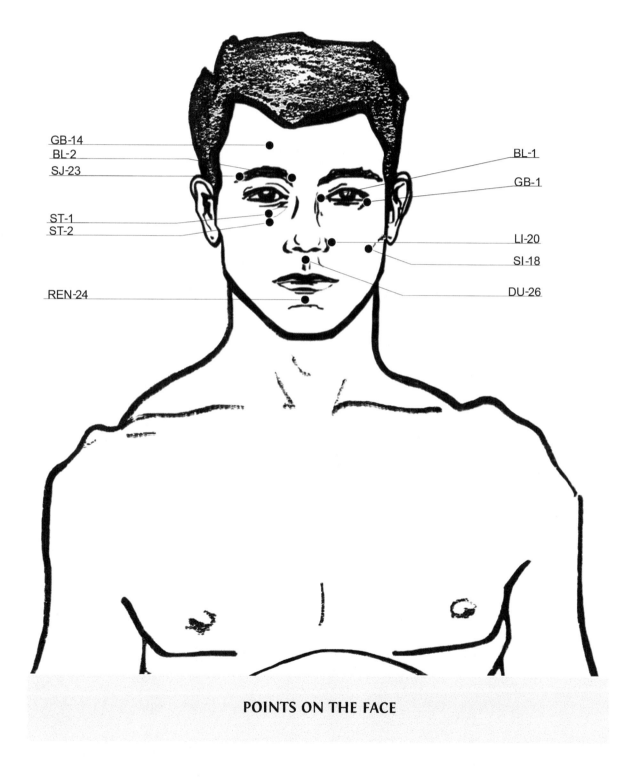

GB-14
BL-2
SJ-23

BL-1

GB-1

ST-1
ST-2

LI-20

SI-18

REN-24

DU-26

POINTS ON THE FACE

151

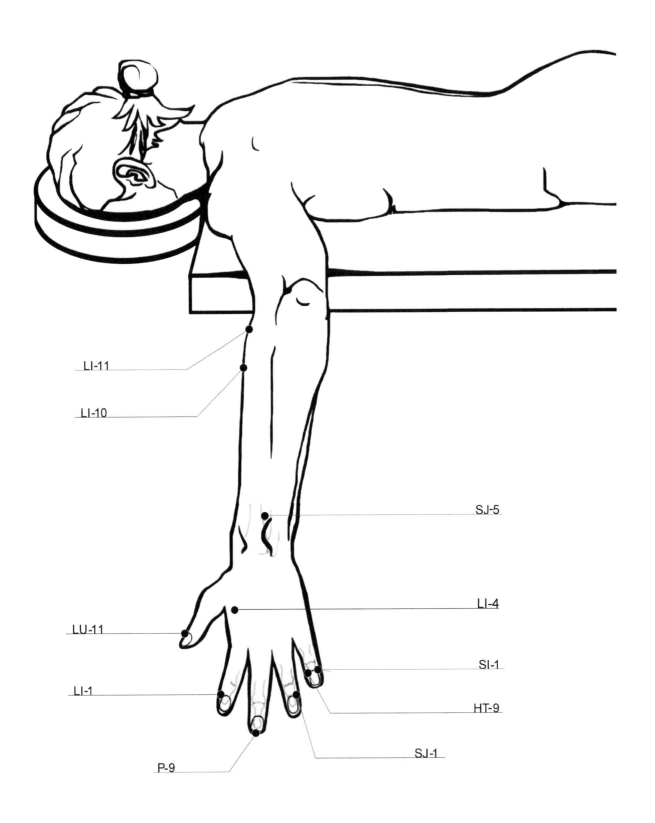

LI-11

LI-10

SJ-5

LI-4

LU-11

SI-1

LI-1

HT-9

SJ-1

P-9

POINTS ON THE POSTERIOR FOREARAM AND HAND

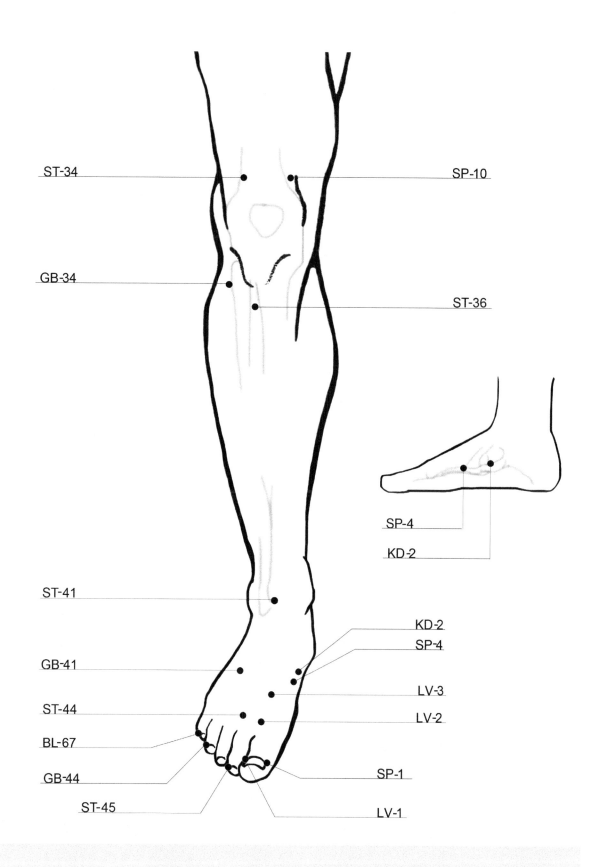

ST-34   SP-10

GB-34

ST-36

SP-4

KD-2

ST-41

KD-2

SP-4

GB-41

LV-3

ST-44

LV-2

BL-67

GB-44

SP-1

ST-45

LV-1

POINTS ON THE FRONT LEG AND FOOT

153

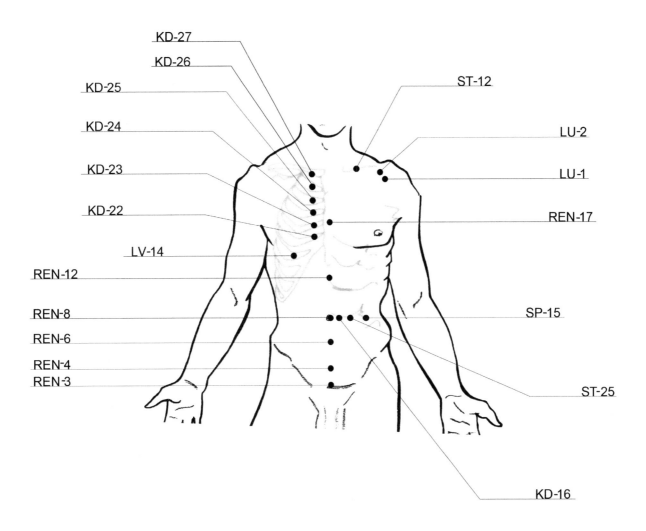

KD-27

KD-26

KD-25

KD-24

KD-23

KD-22

LV-14

REN-12

REN-8

REN-6

REN-4

REN-3

ST-12

LU-2

LU-1

REN-17

SP-15

ST-25

KD-16

POINTS ON THE CHEST AND ABDOMEN

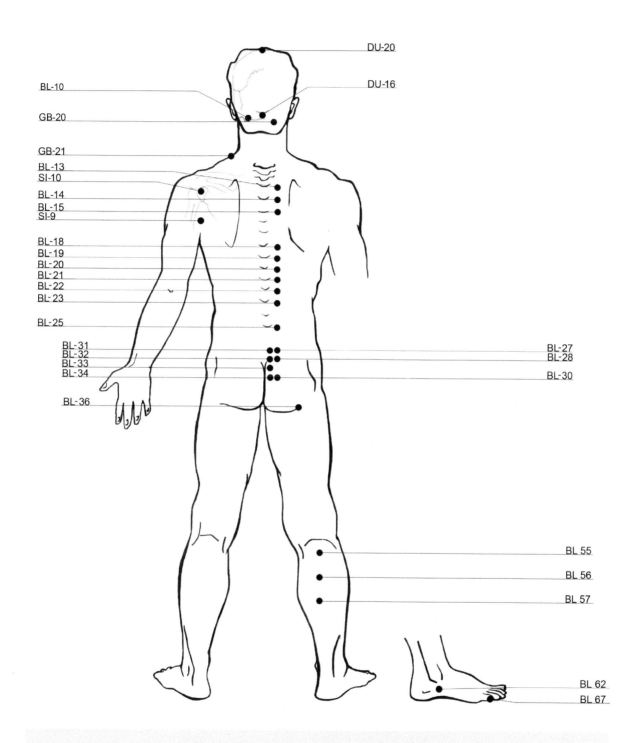

DU-20

DU-16

BL-10

GB-20

GB-21

BL-13

SI-10

BL-14

BL-15

SI-9

BL-18

BL-19

BL-20

BL-21

BL-22

BL-23

BL-25

BL-31

BL-32

BL-33

BL-34

BL-36

BL-27

BL-28

BL-30

BL 55

BL 56

BL 57

BL 62

BL 67

POINTS ON THE BACK OF THE BODY

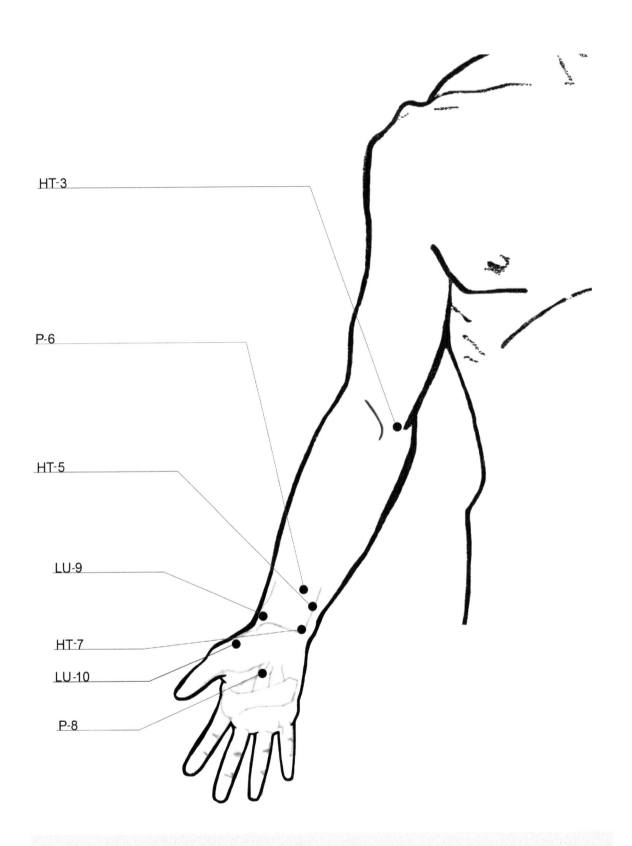

HT-3

P-6

HT-5

LU-9

HT-7

LU-10

P-8

POINTS ON THE ANTERIOR FOREARAM AND HAND

2: The Eight Extraordinary Vessels

There are layers and webs to this energetic medicine. The twelve regular meridians are the pathways for Qi that serve our moment-to-moment needs and can be thought of as one layer. "Underlying" them is what we can think of as a deeper layer, consisting of what are called "extraordinary vessels."

The eight extraordinary vessels are similar to meridians in that Qi flows through them. Yet they are different enough that they are not named "meridians." Only two of these vessels, Du and Ren, have points located on them,

I think of the extraordinary vessels as making up a very deep, behind-the-scenes energetic platform that supports the twelve regular meridians. They often are referred to as reservoirs for Qi. They act both as an "overflow" mechanism to hold an excess of Qi and as a first "place" to pull more Qi from in times of deficiency.

The only meaningful way I have been able to learn about these vessels is to notice what happens when I work on them with clients. Although there are no points on six of the vessels themselves, there are points on meridians that regulate them. These regulation points are called Master Points. The extraordinary vessels are remarkably effective at alleviating energetic imbalances, which is why they must be included in this book. There is not much I can say in words about them, but there is much to learn from experience in the process of using their Master Points.

The eight extraordinary vessels are:

Du (Governing vessel)
Ren (Conception vessel)
Yang Qiao (Yang Heel vessel)
Yin Qiao (Yin Heel vessel)
Yang Wei (Yang Linking vessel)
Yin Wei (Yin Linking vessel)
Dai (Belt vessel)
Chong (Penetrating vessel)

These vessels can be paired within the Yin-Yang duality:

YANG	YIN
Du	Ren
Yang Qiao	Yin Qiao
Yang Wei	Yin Wei
Dai	Chong

The vessels are not, however, associated with either the Five Elements or the Six Channels. In order of their Yin-Yang pairings in the table above, here are some brief descriptions of them and the points associated with them.

"Qi can never be not moving. It is like water flowing, like the sun and the moon traveling without rest. Consequently, the Yin channels nourish the viscera, the Yang channels nourish the bowels. Like a ball without corners, without knowledge of its starting point, the Qi finishes and returns to the beginning." [26]

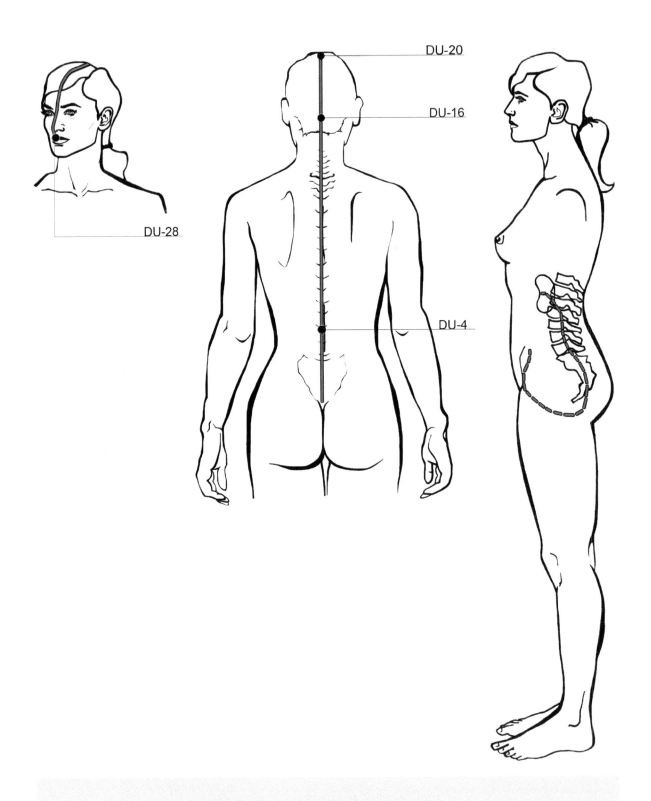

DU-20

DU-16

DU-4

DU-28

THE DU | GOVERNING VESSEL

The Du (Governing) vessel

Yang

Master Point: SI-3

The Du vessel is in charge of all of the Yang meridians of the body.

Primary pathway

The Governing vessel begins in the perineum, enters the coccyx, runs up the sacrum and the spinal column, across the center of the head, down the middle of the forehead, and over the nose to end inside the mouth on the upper gum.

Branches
Branches of the Du enter the brain and kidneys.

Think of the Du when:

Any vertebral, spinal, or brain issues need attention.

Key Du Points (DU-1, 4, 16, 20)

DU-1, Chang Qiang, "Long Strong"

Location: On the perineum just behind the anus.

Use:
This is an important point in the practices of Qi Gong and meditation, not for massage.

DU-4, Ming Men, "Life Gate" or "Door of Life"

Location: Between the spinous process of lumbar vertebrae 2 and 3.
Location tip: Measure from the high point of the posterior iliac crests (the bones of the pelvis) to the vertebrae. This measurement brings you between the fifth and fourth lumbar vertebrae. From this point, feel each spinous process of the lumbar vertebrae, moving up until you are between L2 and L3.

Use:
Being located between the kidneys, where our Life Force literally "sits" in the body, DU-4 is an extremely important point for constitutional vitality—as the Kidneys hold our Essence.

DU-16, Feng Fu, "Palace of Wind"

Location: In the occipital notch.
Location tip: At the base of the skull, even with the vertebral column, locate the occipital notch. It feels like a "soft spot" where the skull meets the upper cervical vertebrae. DU-16 is in this space.

Use:
To open the neck and head to relieve pain and tension
To calm the Spirit

DU-20, Bai Hui, "Hundred Meetings"

Location: In the center of the top of the head, at the highest point.
Location tip: Measure to the center of the head, drawing up from the apex (high point) of the ears to find the point.

Use:
To bring the Qi up
To open the top of the head and let out compressed energy in the head
To relieve headaches
To support concentration and brain function

"Without going outside, you may know the whole world.
Without looking through the window, you may see the ways of heaven.
The farther you go, the less you know.

Thus the sage knows without traveling;
He sees without looking;
He works without doing." [27]

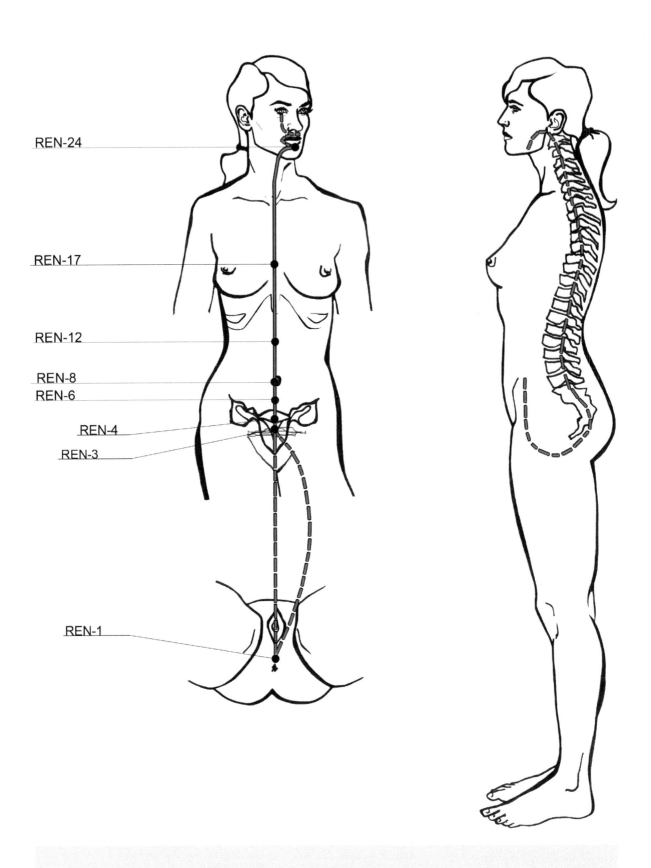

REN-24

REN-17

REN-12

REN-8
REN-6

REN-4

REN-3

REN-1

THE REN | CONCEPTION VESSEL

The Ren (Conception) vessel

Yin

Master Point: LU-7

The Ren vessel governs all of the Yin meridians in the body. The Ren is of primary importance for women as it relates to menstruation, fertility, and pregnancy.

Primary pathway

The primary pathway of the Conception vessel begins in the uterus in women, and in that area in men. It runs up the center of the anterior body to end just below the lower lip on the chin.
Branches

A branch of the Ren runs up the spinal column.

Think of the Ren when:

There are any issues related to menstruation or fertility. Use Ren points to support the production of Blood in menstruating women, to bring the consciousness to the lower abdomen (considered to be one's "energetic center"), and to fortify the Yin.

Key Ren Points (1, 4, 6, 8, 12, 17)

REN-1, Hui Yin, "Meeting of Yin"

Location: On the perineum just in front of the anus and behind the vagina in women and behind the scrotum in men.

Use:
This is an important point in the practices of Qi Gong and meditation, not for massage.

REN-4, Guan Yuan, "Gate of Origin"

Location: 3 cun inferior to the navel.
Location tip: The distance from the navel to the pubic bone is 5 cun. Find REN-4 just a little below the halfway mark between the pubic bone and navel.

This is a very nourishing point for women to support Blood, fertility, the health of the uterus and ovaries.

Use:
To strengthen the Kidney energy, Qi, Blood, Yin and Yang
To help ground the awareness in the abdomen, in the energic center

REN-6, Qi Hai, "Sea of Qi"

Location: 1.5 cun below the navel
Location tip: The width of first and second finger is 1.5 cun. Place these fingers at the lower edge of the navel to locate the point on the center line of the abdomen.

Use:
This is an important point for the male reproductive system and male fertility. Use it
To strengthen Yang and Qi (notice that REN-4 has more Yin function than REN-6).

REN-8, Shen Que, "Spirit Gateway"

Location: The navel.

Use:
This is an important reference point for measuring other Ren points. It is also an important point in Qi Gong and meditation and is considered a "sacred point" of "original nourishment." The navel marks our umbilical cord. The umbilical cord provided the avenue for us to receive nourishment from our birth Mother ("original nourishment") while in her womb. "Sacred" here refers to the reverence we have for this life and the astounding reality that we were originally completely dependent upon our birth Mother and this umbilical cord for growth and development of our body. REN-8 is the navel, which marks our history in the womb.

REN-12, Zhong Wan, "Middle Cavity"

Location: 4 cun superior to the navel.
Location tip: The distance from the navel to the tip of the xiphoid process is 8 cun. REN-12 is halfway between them.

This is an influential point for the Yang Organs.
Use:
For all digestive complaints
To fortify and support all the Yang Organs

REN-17, Shan Zhong, "Chest Center"

Location: In the center of the sternum, level with the fourth intercostal space.

Location tip: The fourth intercostal space is level with the nipples, but the nipples of the breast are not always perfectly at this level, especially as one grows older.

Use:

To disperse the Qi in the chest

To relieve anxiety, panic

To calm the Heart and Spirit

Point combination:

REN-17 + P-6 to calm the Spirit, reduce anxiety.

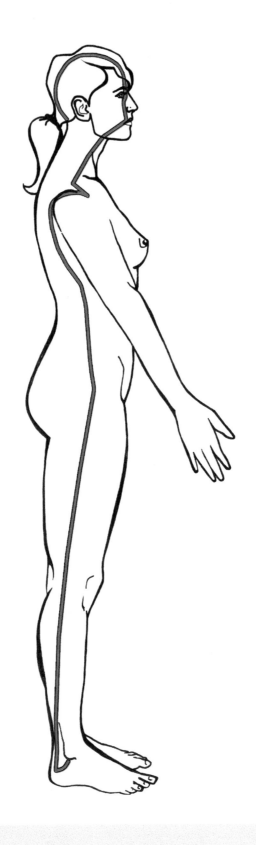

YANG QIAO | YANG MOTILITY VESSEL

Yang Qiao (Yang Heel or Yang Motility) vessel

Yang

Master Point: BL-62

Primary pathway

The Yang Heel vessel starts at the lateral heel, runs up the side of the body, and enters the brain via the outer canthus of the eye. The Yang Qiao is located on both legs and the left and right sides of the body.

Think of the Yang Qiao when:

There is paralysis, or any central nervous system condition. Use it to support the return of activity to the body and mind.

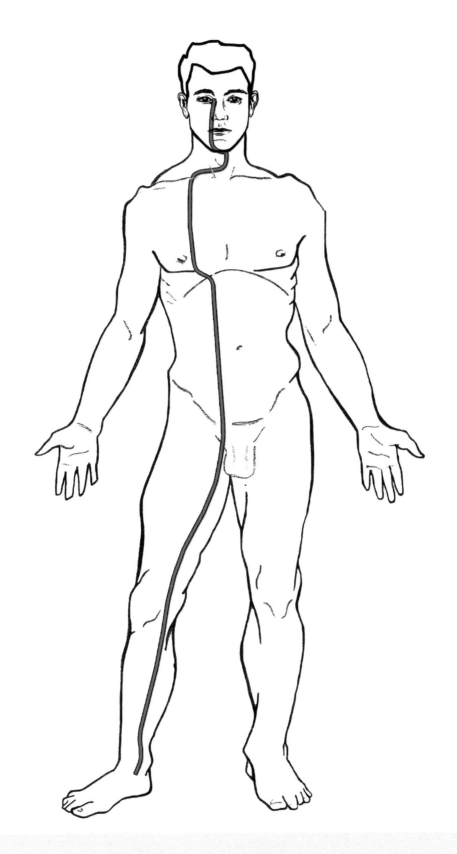

YIN QIAO | YIN MOTILITY VESSEL

Yin Qiao (Yin Heel or Yin Motility) vessel

Yin

Master Point: KD-6

Primary pathway

Yin Qiao starts at the medial heel, runs up the medial leg, abdomen, chest, face, and enters the brain via medial canthus of the eye. The Yin Qiao is located on both legs and the left and right sides of the body.

Think of the Yin Qiao when:

There is paralysis or any central nervous system condition. Use it to nourish the central nervous system deeply.

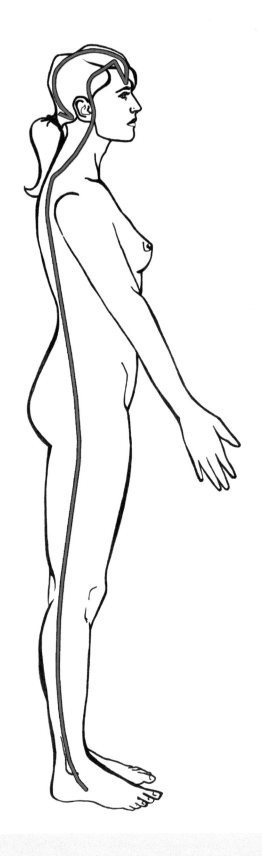

YANG WEI | YANG LINKING VESSEL

Yang Wei (Yang Linking) vessel

Yang

Master Point: SJ-5

Primary pathway

Yang Wei starts at the lateral foot (BL-63), runs up the lateral aspect of the leg and trunk (more posterior to Yang Qiao), covers the side of the head, and ends at DU-16. The Yang Wei is located on both legs and the left and right sides of the body.

Think of the Yang Wei when:

You need to stimulate a general return to activity, a condition of "get up and go," or counteract a mindset of inertia or hopelessness.

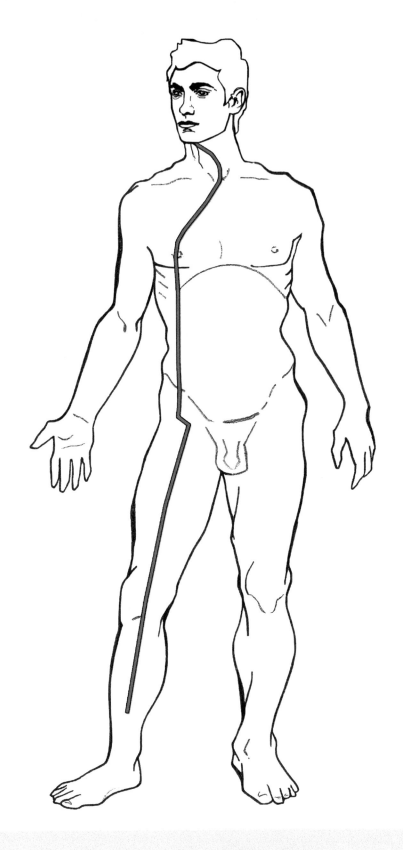

YIN WEI | YIN LINKING VESSEL

Yin Wei (Yin Linking) vessel

Yin

Master Point: P-6

Primary pathway

Yin Wei starts at the medial lower leg, runs up the medial leg, crosses the lateral abdomen and chest, and ends at REN-23 under the chin. The Yin Wei is located on both legs and the left and right sides of the body.

Think of the Yin Wei when:

You need to support a return to deep inner stillness and calm, to direct the awareness inward and toward stillness, or counteract an overactive mindset.

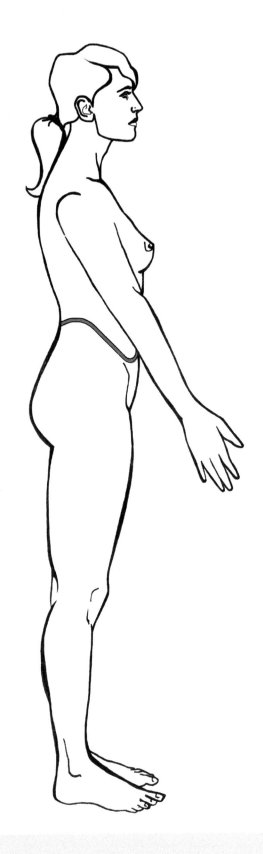

DAI MAI | GIRDLING OR BELT VESSEL

Dai (Belt) vessel

Yang

Master Point: GB-41

Primary pathway

Dai begins in the back, below the ribs at the level of L2 and circles the waist, like a belt.

Think of the Dai when:

You need to energetically reconnect the upper and lower parts of the body.

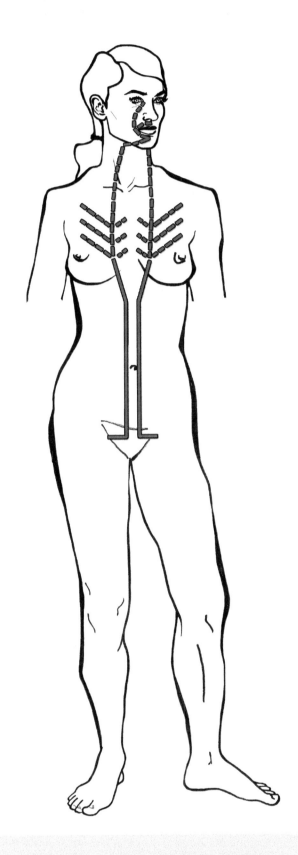

CHONG | PENETRATING VESSEL

Chong (Penetrating) vessel

Yin

Master Point: SP-4

Primary pathway

Chong begins in the lower abdomen (uterus in women), emerges from the lower abdomen and follows the Kidney meridian up the abdomen and chest. Then it disperses further up into the chest, throat, and around the mouth up to the eyes.

Think of the Chong when:

There has been a large loss of blood, as in childbirth or heavy menses. Utilize the Chong vessel to nourish the Blood, as in anemia. If the Blood is weak, it cannot anchor the Mind during sleep, so use the Chong to build Blood to relieve insomnia and the anxious overactive Mind.

Working with the Master Points

I utilize the extraordinary vessels with a broader intention than how I approach the twelve regular meridians. For instance, if a person is in the midst of a crisis, rather than trying to address all the details of the situation I turn to the extraordinary vessels. I find that they can act as a kind of "reset button" for the entire meridian system, bringing a sense of calm, connection, and present-centered awareness.

These vessels are activated by using their Master Points, which are located on the regular meridians and are listed below for each vessel. Practice using combinations of these Points to gain an awareness of how the vessels work. Words are poor descriptors for what they do—experience with them is your best teacher. Below are Master Point combinations used regularly for a variety of common concerns. They offer a solid starting point for you to begin your exploration of the extraordinary vessels.

Master Point combinations

BL-62 + SI-3 – To reduce pain along the vertebral column and neck, and for overall tonifying of Yang. Useful for neck pain specifically when the pain is upon flexion and extension (the nodding "yes" motion).

LU-7 + KD-6 – To activate the Ren and Yin Qiao. Overall nourishment of Yin.

SJ-5 + GB-41 – To reduce pain on the sides of the body, in the hip and shoulder joints, and the neck. Helps with neck pain specifically when the pain is upon rotation from side to side (turning the head side to side, as in the "no" head motion).

SP-4 + P-6 – To calm the Spirit and emotions, to bring inner calm and quiet. Also to fortify and build Blood.

3: Six Channel Theory

As mentioned in Chapter 1 of this section (The Twelve Meridians), the Six Channel perspective is one with which many people in the West are unfamiliar. Basically, it is a way of pairing the meridians according to their positions in the body, so that we work with them in terms of six pairs rather than as twelve individual meridians. It provides a theoretical foundation for seeing and treating how pathogens and disease progress from the exterior to the interior.

Traditionally Six Channel theory has been applied in the context of using herbs in internal medicine, not for external medicine or massage. However, I have found it very beneficial in working with Meridian Massage.

Its Origin

The Six Channel perspective is one of the oldest known organized theories of disease. It is attributed to Zhang Ji, also known as Zhang Zhongjing, the author of the classic Shan Han Lun, "On Cold Damage." He lived and worked as a doctor in China from approximately 150-219 AD, which makes his theory nearly 1800 years old. Zhang Zhongjing holds similar stature in China as Hippocrates does in the West.

Zhang Zhongjing described how external pathogens enter the body, and how the body responds to these invasions. Although thinking of pathogens and the immune system seems natural today, imagine what a breakthrough this was 1800 years ago. The Shan Han Lun offers a coherent and organized system of understanding and evaluating signs, symptoms, and diseases. In addition to this huge breakthrough in medical theory, Zhang Zhongjing describes specific treatments, many of them herbal formulas, to treat conditions arising in each of the six levels or channels this perspective makes available for treatment.

Yin Yang Pairing

Yang is external. Yang provides protection for Yin.

Yin is interior. Yin provides nourishment for Yang.

Of the twelve meridians, six are Yang and six are Yin. By pairing them, we can look at each pair as "one" meridian. The result from this perspective is six meridians (also known as channels) rather than twelve.

When we do this in Six Channel theory, each of the meridians has its same name and functions as it does from the twelve-meridian perspective; here we simply are classifying them differently. Within this classification, certain functions and characteristics stand out more obviously. What stands out makes Six Channel theory a very practical framework for the practice of massage.

Yang covers the posterior and lateral aspects of the body. These areas are more exposed to the elements. Yin covers the anterior and medial aspects of the body. These areas are more protected from the elements.

Feel these differences in your own body. Notice how different the sensations are between touching your abdomen and your back, between your lateral (outer) leg and medial (inner) leg, your anterior (same side as the palm of the hand) forearm and posterior (same side as the back of the hand) forearm, the palm of your hand and the back of your hand. The skin texture and color is different, your emotional responses to being touched are different, your senses of safety and vulnerability are different in these various areas. These differences reflect the different natures of Yin and Yang.

Specific Meridian Pairs in Six Channel theory

The context is that there are six meridians on the leg, and six meridians on the arm. This theory pairs Yang meridians from the arm with Yang meridians from the leg, and Yin meridians from the arm with Yin meridians from the leg. Below is a list of the six channels and the corresponding leg and arm meridians that make up each channel.

Six Channels:

1. Tai Yang (Greater Yang)
    Bladder (leg)
    Small Intestine (arm)

2. Shao Yang (Lesser Yang)
    Gallbladder (leg)
    San Jiao (arm)

3. Yang Ming (Bright Yang)

  Stomach (leg)

  Large Intestine (arm)

4. Tai Yin (Greater Yin)

  Spleen (leg)

  Lung (arm)

5. Shao Yin (Lesser Yin)

  Kidney (leg)

  Heart (arm)

6. Jue Yin (Absolute Yin)

  Liver (leg)

  Pericardium (arm)

The order is given from the most external to the most internal, from "Greater Yang" to "Absolute Yin."

THE SIX CHANNELS	Each of the Six Channels consists of two meridians	
	ARM MERIDIAN	**LEG MERIDIAN**
1. Tai Yang (Greater Yang)	Small Intestine	Bladder
2. Shao Yang (Lesser Yang)	San Jiao	Gallbladder
3. Yang Ming (Bright Yang)	Large Intestine	Stomach
4. Tai Yin (Greater Yin)	Lung	Spleen
5. Shao Yin (Lesser Yin)	Heart	Kidney
6. Jue Yin (Absolute Yin)	Pericardium	Liver

Notice how this ordering progresses from the most exterior (Tai Yang) to the most interior (Jue Yin). From the back (Bladder meridian) to the outer legs and outer arms (SI, SJ, GB, LI, ST) which are more external, we go to the Yin meridians on the inside and medial surfaces of the legs and arms.

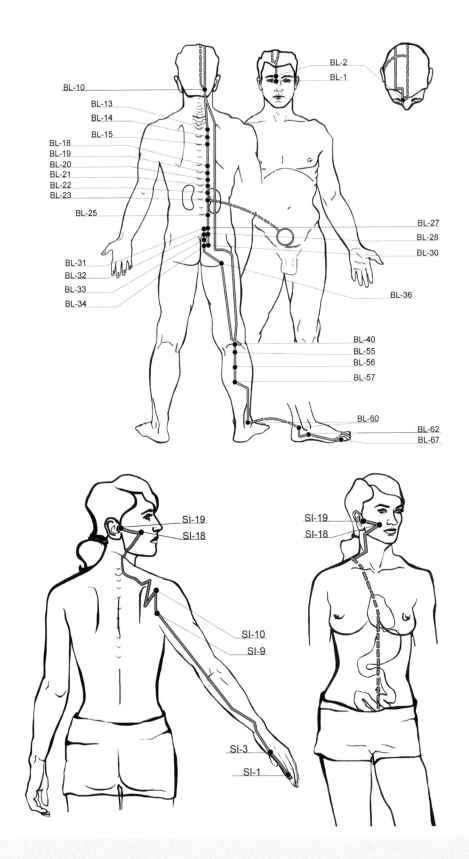

BL-10
BL-13
BL-14
BL-15
BL-18
BL-19
BL-20
BL-21
BL-22
BL-23
BL-25
BL-31
BL-32
BL-33
BL-34
BL-2
BL-1
BL-27
BL-28
BL-30
BL-36
BL-40
BL-55
BL-56
BL-57
BL-60
BL-62
BL-67

SI-19
SI-18
SI-10
SI-9
SI-3
SI-1

TAI YANG (GREATER YANG) | BLADDER (LEG) & SMALL INTESTINE (ARM)

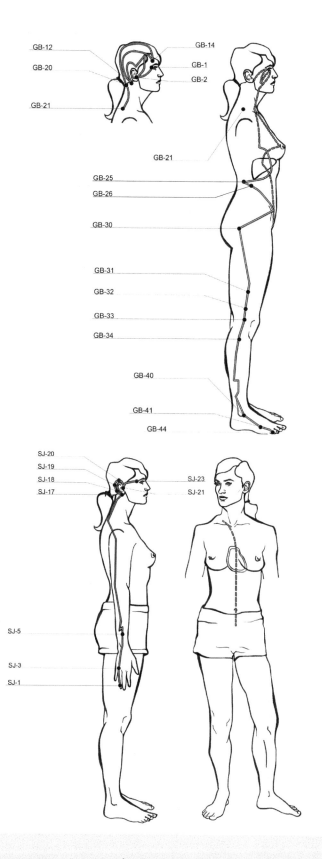

SHAO YANG (LESSER YANG) | GALLBLADDER (LEG) & SAN JIAO (ARM)

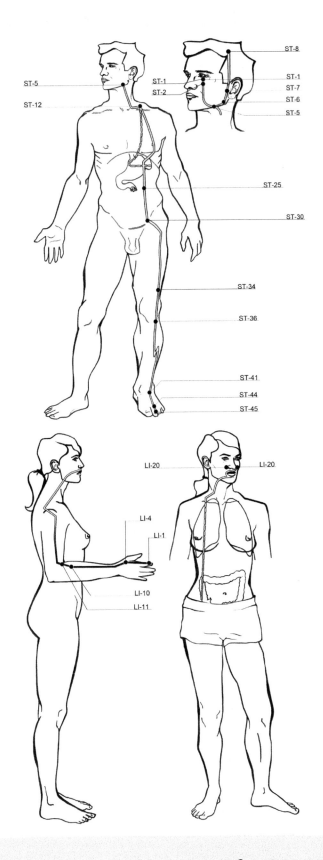

YANG MING (BRIGHT YANG) | STOMACH (LEG) & LARGE INTESTINE (ARM)

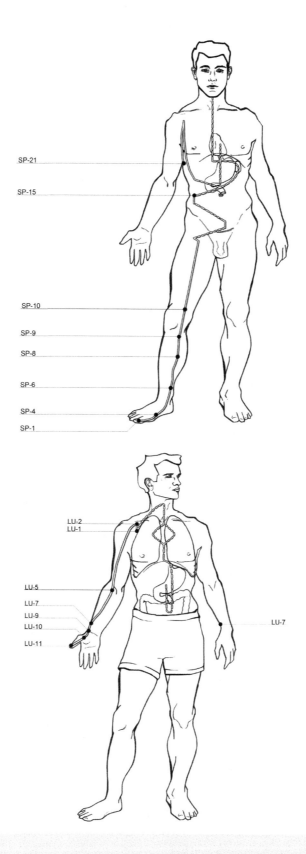

SP-21

SP-15

SP-10

SP-9

SP-8

SP-6

SP-4

SP-1

LU-2
LU-1

LU-5

LU-7

LU-9

LU-10

LU-11

LU-7

TAI YIN (GREATER YIN) | SPLEEN (LEG) & LUNG (ARM)

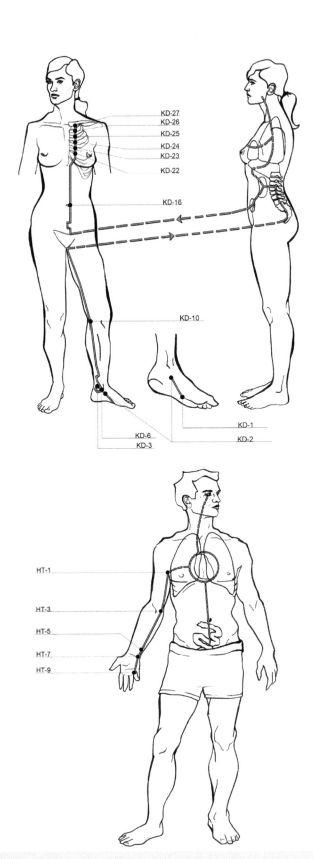

KD-27
KD-26
KD-25
KD-24
KD-23
KD-22

KD-16

KD-10

KD-1
KD-2

KD-6
KD-3

HT-1

HT-3

HT-5

HT-7

HT-9

SHAO YIN (LESSER YIN) | KIDNEY (LEG) & HEART (ARM)

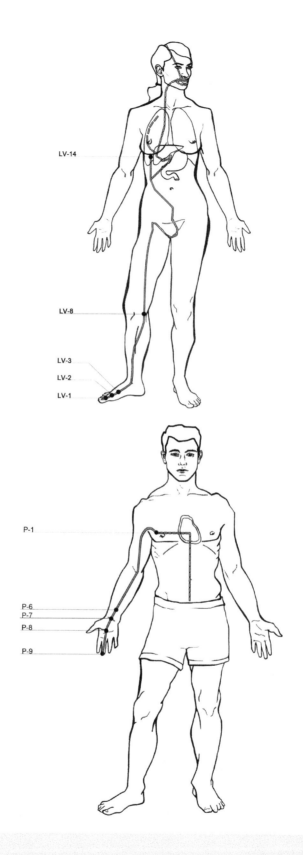

JUE YIN (ABSOLUTE YIN) | LIVER (LEG) & PERICARDIUM (ARM)

Repelling the Invasions of Pathogens

The basic idea is that external pathogens encounter our exterior boundary first. If the pathogen is able to progress inward through the layers of our defenses, the disease gets more serious. The progression from external to internal happens through the meridians.

Meridians are pathways for Qi and for pathogens, just as any street is a pathway for the "good guys" and the "bad guys." External pathogens enter the meridian system from the exterior environment. If the immune system is weak and the pathogen is strong, the pathogen can make its way to the interior. The further into the interior a pathogen goes, the more severe the illness becomes and the more difficult it is to resolve. For example, a stuffy nose (relatively external) is of less concern than pneumonia (relatively internal).

The most exterior meridian (of the six, in this perspective) is the Tai Yang channel, consisting of the bladder and small intestine meridians. The pathological progression of disease is from this most superficial (Tai Yang) layer to the deepest (Jue Yin). The best practitioner prevents disease. The next best practitioner expels the disease from the Tai Yang layer, preventing the progression to the internal organs.

A cold is an example of a disease in the Tai Yang layer. Notice (p. 184) that the early symptoms of a cold match the location of the BL meridian: stiff neck, headache, pain in the forehead.

The external pathogen Wind is commonly the first pathogen into Tai Yang. Wind can block the meridians, which backs up the flow of Qi. The stagnated Qi causes local pain. (See Chapter 2 in Part 3 for more understanding of Bi Syndromes and related external pathogens entering the meridians.) The sources of the "aches and pains" associated with colds and flus are located on the neck and back, bringing stuffy nose, stuffy sinuses. These symptoms reflect blocked BL and SI meridian pathways.

Wind often enters the neck region. Notice (p. 155) that the name of DU-16, at the base of the skull, is Feng Fu, "Palace of Wind." The Lung Shu point (p. 119) is located at T-3 (thoracic vertebrae #3), Fei Shu. At T-2 is the point BL-12, Feng Men, "Wind Gate." These are points where Wind can enter. These points are also used to treat Wind invasions. These are also three good reasons to wear a scarf when out in the wind!

A stiff neck, a headache, a stuffy nose—these are all signs that Wind and Cold have entered the Tai Yang channel (this refers to both the BL and the SI). They can arise quickly after one has been out in the wind and cold or slept near an open breezy window or a fan, or in air conditioning.

Corresponding Western Concept

In Western medicine we speak of microbes, of germs such as bacteria and viruses. Our immune system provides a layer of resistance to these external pathogens. When we have a cold, the symptoms of the cold are actually our body's immune system responding to the rhinovirus (the virus responsible for colds). Holistic Western medicine recognizes the importance of maintaining a healthy immune system to prevent illness.

We may have the experience of catching a cold, ignoring it, and having the situation get worse. At first we had only a stuffy nose, headache, stiff neck and maybe a little fatigue. But a week later we have a sore throat, fever, and exhaustion. The Western practitioner might say now you have strep throat or the flu. The Chinese practitioner might say the pathogen is settling strongly into the Tai Yang layer, and your Yang Defensive Qi is battling pathogenic Qi strongly to avoid further penetration to the Shao Yang layer.

Meridian Massage and the Six Channel Theory

Notice (pp. 194-198) the pathways of Tai Yang, Shao Yang, and Yang Ming. These pathways are common locations of musculoskeletal injury, pain, and restriction. In massage therapy, we are called to attend to these areas more often than to the Tai Yin, Shao Yin, or Jue Yin areas. This is because, as mentioned above, Yang is external and protective of the internal Yin. The Yang meridians, because of their exterior location, are more vulnerable to being invaded by the external pathogens. When these pathogens block the meridians, common symptoms are pain, tension, spasm, or even cramping. (See Chapter 2 in Part 3 for more understanding of Bi Syndromes and related external pathogens entering the meridians.)

The common physical patterns of Qi stagnation that we deal with often show themselves within the Six Channel theory. We can utilize the physical locations of the paired meridians it indicates to better evaluate and treat conditions. Meridian Massage is a hands-on external modality. We are not going to learn in this book how to use herbals and other internal treatments.

Consider, for instance, a condition involving the Shao Yang channel, which consists of the San Jiao (SJ) and Gallbladder (GB) meridians. The client in this case suffers from one-sided headaches (GB), sciatic pain (GB), jaw tension (GB, SJ). Even though most of the symptoms are along the GB meridian, we can utilize the SJ meridian to treat the conditions more effectively. By working the meridians and points along the Shao Yang channel we get better results.

Practitioners who use Meridian Massage from a Western allopathic perspective will encounter the same roadblocks that allopathic medicine encounters regardless of the method of treatment. If you think, in this example, that all one-sided conditions are "classic Gallbladder" symptoms and proceed to only treat the GB meridian, you will have missed an essential aspect of what Chinese medicine makes available.

As we know from earlier chapters, the meridians are part of a whole web of pathways in/through which Qi travels. As is so for each meridian, the Gallbladder meridian in this example must be understood in its larger context. The GB meridian is the Shao Yang partner of San Jiao and the Wood Yang partner of the Liver.

Now let's revisit the client with one-sided headaches, jaw pain, and sciatica.

The GB meridian traverses the side of the head, the jaw, and the hip. This is a classic pattern of Qi stagnation in the GB meridian. But notice also that the SJ meridian is on the side of the head, tucked in more closely behind the ear. Now is a good time ask about ear issues: any pain or stuffiness in the ear?

There are three points located over the temporal mandibular joint: SI-19, SJ-21, GB-2. Again we see the GB–SJ connection. GB-30 is the point right on the area where the piriformis muscle crosses the sciatic nerve. So we begin to see that if we want to clear the GB meridian, we may get a better result if we clear out both of the SJ and the GB.

I also mentioned that GB is the Yang meridian of the Wood Element. What does the Liver have to do with these conditions? The Liver is in charge of keeping the Qi moving smoothly throughout the body. Any Qi stagnation in any meridian points to stagnation in the Liver. What stagnates the Liver? Toxicity. What is toxicity? Nasty food, drugs (prescribed or not), alcohol, and sedentary living are lifestyle realities that mess with the Liver. In any condition it is also important to consider if internal pathogens are present. These "pathogens" are the negative emotions associated with a given Element. For Wood, we have anger and frustration as two associated internal pathogens. Is the client angry, or frustrated?

Wood energy is growing, expanding, moving, inspiring, bursting forth—just like springtime. When we are not able to express our big selves, when we feel there is not enough room for, or acceptance of, our genuine self, we hold ourselves back, keep cool, rein it in. This action creates a very strong energetic block to the movement of our Qi, the Qi stagnates, and symptoms arise. Besides headaches, sciatica, etc., stagnated Liver Qi symptoms include appearing to be a very tense high-strung person (he/she has a ton of energy within that isn't being allowed to come out), a bouncing knee, being always in a rush, speaking sharply, being prone to angry outbursts when no longer able to contain oneself.

Imagine trying to hold back the sprouting tulips, the gushing water from melting ice in spring, the birth of a child. What might this look like in a person?

What does the "superior healer" do for a client with all these symptoms? We try to apply the same intention regardless of the person and their symptoms. We want to support and encourage the smooth and harmonious flow of Qi throughout their whole body-mind-spirit. In this case, we need to move Qi in the GB, SJ, and Liver meridians. Simultaneously we encourage shifts in lifestyle that support the flow of Qi, that soothe the Liver, and inspire the authentic expression of the client's true self.

In Six Channel theory the Liver is paired with Pericardium. The point P-6 is the command point of the chest. Stress, frustration, and containment often bring about shallow breathing, which contributes to Qi gathering and stagnating in the chest. There is a sense of fullness in the chest, of there not being enough in the space in the body, of pressure. We can use the point combination of REN-17 + P-6 to calm the Heart and Spirit, and to descend the Qi in the chest.

The meridians are a web of inter-relating pathways. Combining the pairings from the Six Channel Theory with the pairings in Five Element Theory reveals another layer of relationship among them. As you can see from just the brief example above, Six Channel perspective makes information available that may be hard to discover without it.

For more detail, consider the pairings below:

In the vertical columns we see pairings from the Six Channel perspective—for example Bladder/ Small Intestine as one pair and Kidney/Heart as another. In the horizontal rows we see pairings from the Five Element perspective—Bladder/Kidney as one pair, and Intestine/Heart as another.

	6 Channel Pair	6 Channel Pair
	Tai Yang	Shao Yang
Water Element	BLADDER	KIDNEY
Fire Element	SMALL INTESTINE	HEART

	6 Channel Pair	6 Channel Pair
	Shao Yang	Jue Yin
Wood Element	GALLBLADDER	LIVER
Fire Element	SAN JIAO	PERICARDIUM

	6 Channel Pair	6 Channel Pair
	Yang Ming	ShaoYin
Earth Element	STOMACH	SPLEEN
Metal Element	LARGE INTESTINE	LUNG

Seeing these deeper connections between meridians creates an opportunity to get underneath the superficial symptoms of muscle and joint pain. We are better informed as to how to get to the root-causes of patterns that repeatedly give rise to the same issue in different areas of the body, or at different times in one's life.

In my work as a massage therapist, I have often felt that I was missing some deeper connections to my client's issues. As much as I appreciated being able to relieve their pain while we were together, the pain usually came back. Then I began to notice that many musculoskeletal issues are found on the Tai Yang, Shao Yang, and Yang Ming channels.

Finding connections between the Six Channel pairs and the Five Element pairs opens an avenue for deeper investigation into hidden patterns that allow or provoke chronic surface patterns of muscle tension and joint pain at one level, and that, at a deeper level cause plenty of limitation and suffering in their own right.

To address the deep root patterns, we have to address the internal pathogens—the negative emotions. These patterns are harder to access and harder to clear up. It's commonly said in Chinese medicine that emotions injure the Organs. This is no metaphor, it's a real phenomenon.

So for the person in the example above, the pattern of excess frustration and anger in response to circumstances overtaxes the Liver. Over time the Liver becomes stagnated and irritated, leading to stagnation in the all of the meridians in general but in the Gallbladder in particular. So now she comes for bodywork to get help relieving sciatic pain or jaw tension.

Opening the meridians and moving the Qi will quite easily alleviate those symptoms, but not the underlying pattern of Liver Qi stagnation that sets the stage for these ailments in the first place. We have to go deeper, to the Organs themselves, to address that. And this is what brought me to the study of abdominal massage.

The meridians are "branches" that lead out from Organs. Clearing up meridians is part of the puzzle we work with, yes. But clearing up the Organs is like pulling out the bottom card in a stack of cards—all the superficial issues come crashing down. So to have a chance at real and permanent change, rather than only chasing stagnation through the meridian system, we need to also address the challenges at the deeper level.

When we contact the abdominal Organs, we touch right into the center of the person—right into the Organs that have been absorbing, processing, and holding Qi. It is here in the Organs that we can help our clients address their negative internal pathogens—emotions and mental habits that keep them in patterns that limit them physically, emotionally, mentally, and spiritually.

Each human being is a single unit that combines many aspects: mind, physical, spiritual, emotional, energetic, material. Real change that affects all of these levels is possible. We practitioners can help clients with this type of transformation by combining our use of the meridian system with massage to the abdominal Organs.

See Part 3, Chapter 3, for details on abdominal massage.

4: Yuan Source Points

These are specific points for contacting "Source Qi." Source Qi refers to the Qi of our Life Force. The Kidneys hold the Essence or "Life Force." All Qi is precious, but I think of this Source Qi as "extra precious."

Water, like Qi, is vital to life. Imagine the Qi in the meridians as water moving along streams. Now imagine our water system today. Many of us drink "city water" which is pumped to us from a central city source.

This still is water, and it is vital to our health. But . . .

Have you ever had water from a deep, pristine well? Or from a spring that is pure, clear, and drawing right from the source? This kind of water tastes and feels very different than "regular" water. Touching into Yuan Source points is like accessing the purest water from a pristine source.

Yuan source points are found on all twelve meridians. The points on Yin meridians are particularly potent points for nourishing the related Organ. Following this line of thought, the Kidney source point is of utmost importance (because the Kidney is the Yin Organ of the Water Element).

Yin Organs hold, transform, and maintain our Qi, Essence, Blood—all things necessary for life. Use Yin meridian Source points to bring the freshest, purest Qi to the related Organ. I use them to revitalize and nourish the energy of exhausted people, to maintain the energy of people under high stress, people undergoing surgery or chemotherapy, and people recovering from long-term illnesses.

Yang source points do not have the same nourishing properties as the Yin source points. While the table on the opposite page lists both the Yin and the Yang points, in practice I use only the Yin source points for the purposes stated above.

YUAN SOURCE POINTS, PAIRED BY YIN AND YANG

YIN MERIDIANS	YANG MERIDIANS
KD-3: Tai Xi, "Supreme Stream"	BL-64: Jing Gu, "Capital Bone"
LV-3: Tai Chong, "Great Rushing"	GB-40: Qiu Xi, "Mound of Ruins"
SP-3: Tai Bai, "Supreme White"	ST-42: Chong Yang, "Rushing Yang"
LU-9: Tai Yuan, "Supreme Abyss"	LI-4: He Gu, "Joining Valley"
P-7: Da Ling, "Great Mound"	SJ-4: Yang Chi, "Yang Pool"
HT-7: Shen Men, "Spirit Gate"	SI-4: Wan Gu, "Wrist Bone"

5: Ma Dan Yang Heavenly Star Points

Ma Dan Yang was a famous practitioner in twelfth-century China. He gathered a group of eleven acupoints that he considered to be the most important points. Another accomplished physician, Xu Feng, later added a twelfth to this group. This group of points has come to be known as Ma Dan Yang's Heavenly Star Points. Because Ma Dan Yang was so famous his set of points remains as a core of very important points. The Heavenly Star Points are very potent and should be known by all practitioners.

Ma Dan Yang Heavenly Star Points - AKA 12 Heavenly Star Points

LU-7	BL-40
LI-4	BL-57
LI-11	BL-60
HT-5	GB-30
ST-36	GB-34
ST-44	LV-3

6: Master Points

The extraordinary vessels other than Du and Ren do not have any points. Each vessel can be activated by using a specific point on one of the twelve regular meridians. These points are called "Master Points."

The Master Points for each extraordinary vessel are as follows:

MASTER POINT	AREA OF BODY
SI-3	Du
BL-62	Yang Qiao
LU-7	Ren
KD-6	Yin Qiao
SJ-5	Yang Wei
GB-41	Dai Mai
P-6	Yin Wei
SP-4	Chong

Master Point Combinations

There are many possible combinations of Master Points. Here are some commonly used combinations and the indication for each combination:

SI-3 + BL-62: Overall muscle pain, back pain.

LU-7 + KD-6: Lung issues, nourishes overall Yin of body.

SJ-5 + GB-41: Side of the body, neck pain, opens GB meridian as a whole, one sided issues.

P-6 + SP-4: Chest and Heart issues, women's reproduction, calming and quieting. This combination is brings attention inward.

In practice I often use only one or two of these combinations. However, I have found that the best way to learn about these combinations is to give and receive a session using just these combinations. Hold the points on one side of the body and then switch to the other. Hold each combination for at least three breaths and then let your intuition guide you from there.

7: Command Points

A "Command Point" is a point we use to direct the Qi to a specific area of the body. In practice, these points are used as general way to "guide" or "focus" all of the work done in a session to a particular area. For example, if the client has neck pain, use LU-7 to direct all of your efforts toward that area.

Here is a list of them and the areas to which they direct Qi:

COMMAND POINT	AREA OF BODY
LU-7	Neck and Head
LI-4	Face and Mouth
ST-36	Abdomen
BL-40	Lower Back (upper also, but famous for lower)
P-6	Chest and Heart

8: Point Combinations

In practice, we use points in combination. I combine points with other points, I alternate contacting points and the associated meridian, and I combine points with the associated Organ. Do not limit yourself to the combinations listed here, but do experiment with them as they are traditional combinations handed down over hundreds of years.

Classic Combinations

LI-4 + LV-3: Moves Qi of the whole body

ST-36 + ST-44: Useful for all GI issues

BL-40 + BL-57: For low back pain

GB-30 + GB-34: For lumbar pain, any spasm anywhere, one-sided pain and tension, any motor impairment.

Combinations with Command Points

ST-36 + ST-25 + SP-15: For abdominal pain, digestion issues

P-6 + REN-17: For anxiety, palpitations, insomnia

SP-6 + REN-3, 4, 6: For female reproductive issues, urinary tract infection

BL-40 + BL-23: For low back pain

LI-4 + ST-44: For tooth abscess

" The key to mastering health is to regulate the yin and the yang of the body. If the yin and yang balance is disrupted, it is like going through a year with spring but no winter, or winter but no summer. When the yang is excessive and cannot contain itself, the yin will become consumed. Only when the yin remains calm and harmonious will the yang qi be contained and not overly expansive, the spirit normal, and the mind clear." [28]

Part 3

Hands-On Meridian Massage

1: Treatment Principles

Hands-on Meridian Massage is a process of applying seven basic principles:

1. Balance Yin and Yang.

2. Encourage/support communication and harmony between Fire and Water, Heart and Kidney.

3. Support the flow of Qi from top to bottom and bottom to top.

4. Support the flow of Qi from the center to the extremities, and the extremities to the center.

5. Support the flow of Qi from the interior to the exterior, and the exterior to the interior.

6. Balance movement and stillness.

7. Facilitate meeting points.

1. Balance Yin and Yang

Balancing Yin and Yang is the basis of this work. All other principles are permutations of how to balance Yin and Yang. Balance requires communication between Yin and Yang. We need to know how each moves individually and how they move as partners.

Yin nourishes Yang, Yang protects Yin. This spontaneous inter-activity is a living, organic motion. If there is not enough Yin to nourish the Yang, Yang will not have an anchor and will tend to rise and scatter. If there is not enough Yang to protect the Yin, Yin is exposed and open to leakage and decrease.

When Yin and Yang are communicating and moving well, the physical manifestations are ease, flexibility, flow, contentment, satisfaction, and health. We then have more conscious awareness of our inner resources and therefore more opportunity to envision and live the life we dream in our hearts. Night becomes day, day becomes night. Frustration becomes fortitude and perseverance. Fear becomes presence and peace.

If we resist our emotions, we resist the natural motion from one energetic/emotional state to the next: We literally resist the movement of Yin and Yang. This resistance creates stagnation. Stagnation prevents the flow of Qi and reinforces unconscious perspectives and behaviors that continue the cycle of stagnation.

Energetic/emotional stagnation will manifest physically as groups of signs and symptoms that are then labeled as a certain disease. Points where the stagnation builds up interrupt the flow of Qi and become places of non-communication between Yin and Yang, mind and body, conscious and unconscious. We then need "inner work" to reconnect our conscious awareness with these places and unravel the energetic knot/stagnation.

Our focus always is to support the balance of Yin and Yang.

2: Encourage/support communication and harmony of Fire and Water, Heart and Kidney

Yin-Water and Yang-Fire manifest in the human body as the Organs Heart (Fire) and Kidney (Water). To know our Heart is to literally touch into Yang. To know our Kidneys is to literally touch into Yin.

Balance Fire and Water by using the Fire and Water meridians. Choose point combinations from these two meridians that support the interaction and communication of these two primary forces.

Water and Fire are the extremes of Yin and Yang. At the highest peak of Yang, the energy will transform into Yin. At lowest extreme of Yin, the energy will transform into Yang. These are the extreme changes, the big fluctuations, big crises, big symptoms.

Recall that the Heart houses the Spirit. Mental-emotional concerns have to do with the balance (or imbalance, non-communication) between Fire and Water, Heart and Kidneys. Too much heat will literally dry up the fluids (Yin). As this drying continues, Yang will lose its root, its source of nourishment (Yin Water). In this state, the Heart is no longer a stable, calm home for the Spirit (Shen).

Imagine the Shen (Spirit) as the flame of a candle. The flame is grounded by the wick and fueled by the wax. As the wax dwindles, the flame grows large and flickers wildly—just before going out. This is like a "rootless Shen" or a floating mind unable to get grounded within its body.

The Mind must rest in the Blood at night. Yin is supposed to overtake Yang at night, so that we sleep. If the Yin is too weak, it cannot take over the Yang and we don't sleep. If the Blood (Yin) is deficient (has gotten burned off from too much Fire), then the Mind has no place to rest. At night this person is unable to fall asleep, or wakes up during the night, or has bad dreams.

When is the last time you gazed in awe at a candle without a flame? With not enough Yang, we lose our brightness, our shine, our get-up-and-go, our warmth. It's similar when our Yang has decreased too much relative to our Yin, creating imbalance. The person with this pattern is often chilly or cold (not enough Fire), sluggish, tired, unmotivated.

When the inspiration of Yang is overpowered by the excess amount of Yin, not much is happening because the force of movement and Yin is the force of stillness. Then, just as we cut away excess wax when it floods the flame we have to drain off the excess Yin fluids and call the Yang back in. When the Yang returns and establishes a better balance with Yin, heat, warmth, movement, and motivation also return.

3: Support the flow of Qi from top to bottom and bottom to top

If you spend a lot of time working the head, neck, and shoulders, be sure to work the legs, ankles, and feet as well. The Qi that is released from all the work up above needs a place to flow. Open up the lower areas to allow that Qi a place to go.

In the West, up is judged as "good." We tend to easily bring our attention and energy up. Modern Western-minded people need extra help bringing Qi down. When the Qi is penned in above, help guide it down to enliven the lower body and relieve pressure in the upper areas.

Alternatively, if you spend a lot of time working on the abdomen, hips, legs, and feet, open up the chest, arms, head, and neck as well. The Qi that you awaken in the lower body and lower extremities will want to move. Create space in the chest, arms, neck, and head for it to move up.

Opening the upper body and head is like taking the lid off a steaming pot. As the Qi gets moving, it wants to flow. If you don't take the lid off, the pot will rattle and shake from the built-up pressure. If you don't open your client's upper body and extremities, it is likely that the unconscious patterns of containing the Qi will return. Opening meridian pathways relieves the pressure of containing the Qi in one small space.

Moving Qi requires creating space for it to flow. On the table, your clients may experience this flowing Qi and enjoy it. Even better is to ensure the continuation of this flow when they return to their life. To facilitate this, help your clients become very consciously aware of what feels different in their body as you work with them. Try asking, "What's different? What does this open, flowing, moving, harmonized Qi feel like?" We want that to become the new "unconscious normal" setting in the body.

Many people have become habituated to living in a body that is out of balance, with places of energetic stagnation. If we do not bring this open, flowing state to their conscious awareness while they are in it, their habituated body-mind may construe the return to flow and "real balance" as "out of balance." When we do not consciously take time to reorient the person to true balance and flow, the habituated body-mind often swiftly reconstructs the tension patterns that we just adjusted, and unconscious tension patterns that were holding back the Qi return.

The return to tension can be very uncomfortable, as it seems to the habit pattern that the muscles have to work twice as hard to get things back to "normal" from this place of more motion and openness. The "reconstruction" can manifest as painful muscle spasms that restrict movement of the physical body and the flow of Qi in the meridians. Often the return is not so drastic as acute cramping, but still, the pattern returns and the client remains limited by the stagnation.

What results from this process is a person who keeps coming for bodywork—the person is able to get some relief on your table yet not able to maintain the changes in everyday life. To actually maintain the changes in Qi flow, the client will have to consciously participate to preserve the changes you introduce during the hands-on session. They need to learn how to make adjustments in their lifestyle and mindset that support the free flow of Qi rather than to recreate the habitual tension patterns set up around points of Qi stagnation. Sometimes these adjustments are small and subtle. Sometimes they call for big life changes.

4: Support the flow of Qi from the center to the extremities, and the extremities to the center

Massaging the abdomen is a profound way to support the movement of Qi between the Organs. Take breaks from working intently in the center to contact the extremities. Make sure the shoulders and inguinal (lower pelvic) areas are open to allow the flow between the extremities and the center.

Imagine the abdomen as the ocean and the head and extremities as tributaries. Keep the joints open, the meridians open, to allow Qi to move in and out of the center to the extremities.

The extremities draw their Qi from the center. To ensure proper nourishment and flow to the extremities, be sure to touch into the abdomen even when working on meridians and points located on the extremities. Friction to the tips of all the fingers, toes, and Kidney 1 on the sole of the foot is a quick and effective way to activate Qi flow in all twelve meridians.

Again, take time to bring your client's conscious attention to the changes—the feeling of openness and the ease of unimpeded Qi flow. The conscious mind must be convinced that everything is okay even with all this Qi flowing. Take care to maintain the client's sense of safety, so as to keep the protective fight-or-flight response from flipping on and restoring the pattern of tension that held the Qi in stagnation.

5: Support the flow of Qi from the interior to the exterior, and the exterior to the interior

The interior is Yin, the exterior is Yang. We encourage the dance and communication of Yin and Yang by balancing our deep work with our superficial strokes.

Coach your clients to sense their interior world by following the feeling of their breath into their lungs, the movement of their chest and belly as the breath moves. Keep bringing their inner awareness to their interior structures such as organs, bones, muscles, and other areas with your pressure and verbal cues. This is how we literally help people feel their way into their inner world.

Feeling one's own Qi is challenging. You help your clients learn how to sense their Qi by helping them bring their attention inward and develop the skill of feeling for their Qi. Doing this can seem very esoteric to them, or out of the range of their reality—which is why it is imperative for us therapists to learn to feel our own Qi. Only your actual experience of sensing your Qi will make you able to help others feel theirs.

Again, Yin is interior, Yang is exterior. The skill of moving attention from Yin interior to Yang exterior develops over time through practice. This skill helps us integrate Yin and Yang.

6: Balance movement and stillness

Return to simplicity. Yang is motion, Yin is stillness. Modulate your work between stillness and movement. Invite your clients to take part in this by asking them to move at appropriate times, as in breathing deeply or even moving limbs gently. Invite them to stillness by inviting them to be quiet and listen internally to the call of their center.

Move the Qi with more vigorous strokes. Quiet and consolidate it with still holds, slower motion, and your own quiet attention.

7: Facilitate meeting points

For the work to have lasting value, your client must experience balance, harmony, and flow on a regular basis. Opening Qi flow means that something has to melt, move, disintegrate within the meridians. Often the block is emotionally based—something that keeps the information, memory, sensations of the Organ, meridian, or area away from consciousness.

These are vulnerable and challenging places. Yet, if Qi is going to flow and allow Yin and Yang to balance, what I call a "meeting point" must be established and communication opened there. We facilitate bringing attention inward to these precise points where resistance, density, pain, or numbness are. These are the places that require attending to. They are the precise location(s) of the blocked meridian and the stagnation.

When attention comes to the location of stagnation, we have a meeting point. A meeting point is the place/moment of conscious mind meeting unconscious energetic block—when the client becomes consciously aware of and sensitive to the previously unconscious block.

Unconscious blocks do not just disappear. They have to be made conscious. They have to be opened by the collaboration of the therapist's skill and the client's ability to consciously let them go. When a meeting point is established and helped/allowed to open, Qi flows, information flows, and the energetic web of meridians can rebalance.

Our "work" is to facilitate the journey inward to the meeting points and to be present with or witness to the communication that happens there. It is also to stay out of the way as the energetic mending proceeds.

Summary

As I never tire of saying, getting to "simple" can be a complicated process. The simple intention of Meridian Massage is to balance Yin and Yang and support the free flow of Qi. We use the dynamics of Yin and Yang to guide the work. Yin and Yang are complementary opposites, just like inner and outer, up and down, motion and stillness.

Being present with a person who is engaging a meeting point continues to be moving and inspiring to me. It takes courage, perseverance, patience, and trust to consciously seek the source of our energetic blocks, as these places are often sites of deep emotional, mental, spiritual, or physical pain. In these sacred meeting places, things really can and do change.

2: Obstruction Syndromes – "Bi Syndromes"

The word "Bi" in Chinese means obstruction. Bi Syndromes are a particular kind of Qi blockage. Chinese medicine attributes joint pain and arthritis to them, also chronic tendonitis, muscle spasms, and cramps. Bi Syndromes are active in trigger points or "knots" in the muscles where there is a block in the meridian and the Qi cannot flow. As the Qi backs up at the site of the obstruction (stagnation), we feel distention, pain, tenderness. Over time, chronic Qi stagnation can manifest as more severe physical conditions such as deformation of joints.

Regardless of where these Syndromes are, their underlying cause is the same: The meridian is obstructed, the Qi is stagnated, pain is the result. Massage is a practical and direct method of treatment often used to clear Bi Syndromes.

As mentioned earlier, one of the things I appreciate most about the Chinese medical approach is that by addressing the underlying Qi, many different manifestations can be cleared up at once. There are many possible manifestations of energetic imbalances and many different ways to address them—some better than others. If I chase trigger points, arthritis, and tendonitis as separate conditions, for example, I'll be chasing them for a long time. And that is what I did for many years before learning about Bi Syndromes.

Understanding Bi Syndromes is very helpful for assessing a client's situation, because they account for external causes of pain and tension often overlooked by modern medicine. That understanding also helps guide your hands-on working sessions.

I have noticed that Bi Syndromes arise mostly along Yang meridians. Yang is more external and exposed to factors present in the conditions of our physical climate.

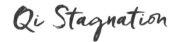

Qi Stagnation

Block in the meridian

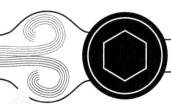

Example of a Meridian

Qi backs up in the meridian
= STAGNATION. Feels like:
pain, distension, frustration

Direction of Qi flow

What blocks the meridians?

Musculoskeletal pain is most often due to stagnated Qi. The meridians are the pathways where the Qi flows. If there is a block in the meridian, the Qi cannot flow.
There are three categories of blockages:

1. Trauma, such as slamming your toe into a hard unmovable object.
2. External pathogens, such as Wind, Cold, Damp, Heat.
3. Internal pathogens, such as the emotions of fear, anger, anxiety, sadness, worry, grief, and overexcitement.

Bi Syndromes are in the second category, blockage caused by external pathogens. Limbs, muscles, and joints are external (as compared to organs which are internal). Bi Syndromes affect the meridians and structures that cover the external surfaces. To address the Bi Syndromes, we focus on the external pathogens using external interventions, such as massage, acupuncture, or applications of heat or cold.

Four Types of Bi Syndromes

There are four types of Bi Syndromes:

1. *Wind.* Pain moves around, just like the wind. "First my neck hurts, then my elbow, now it seems to be back in my neck."

2. *Cold.* Severe pain located in a specific spot is often cold to the touch. "My hip is killing me, no matter what position I'm in, it still hurts!"

3. *Damp.* Pain severity is between Wind and Cold, swelling at the location, and the pain lingers. "My elbow is puffy and sore, it hasn't gone away in a week."

4. *Heat.* Pain is severe, acute, and hot. This usually only happens in hot, humid months and is less common than the other three Bi Syndromes.

These pathogens are also climatic factors. Science tends to deny these factors as "old wives' tales." But experience shows us that the old wives were wise, not foolish. In the West, we are used to putting on a coat in chilly weather to avoid "catching a cold." Even though some modern theories insist that we get colds from germs, not from the temperature, common sense and experience show us that being out in the cold creates the condition of a "cold."

Expand this perspective to include Wind, Damp, Heat—it's that simple. These climatic factors can penetrate the boundaries of our skin and meridians. When they enter the meridian system they disrupt the flow of Qi, which creates symptoms. "Put on your jacket or you might catch a wind."

Wind is very good at penetrating our meridian system, which is why people in the East are much more mindful of staying out of the wind than we are in the West. Wind often opens the gate for the Cold and Damp to enter. Need experiential learning? Go stand on the beach in Maine in April for an hour or two (without your coat, hat, and mittens) and you will experience Wind, Cold, and Damp penetrating your barriers and entering your meridian system.

For our purposes, we don't need to spend time deciphering which individual pathogen is the biggest player. The obstruction is most likely caused by a combination of all three. One of the pathogens will become obvious at some point during the treatment.

If the main pathogen is Cold, add heat to your treatment. If it is Damp, add drying heat. If it is Wind, just get it out. But don't add heat to a Heat Bi! Don't be paranoid, but just don't put a heat lamp or hot stones or hot water bottle on a red, inflamed, hot, painful joint in the middle of summer!

Differences in manifestation and severity

Who is the person with you right now, with the pain you want to address? This matters! Is the person twenty-five or fifty-five or seventy-five or ninety-five? How long has the obstruction been there? Is it in the muscles, tendons, or joints? If joints, which joints—knee, shoulder, cervical vertebrae? Is the person active or sedentary? Are they interested in what they can do or change to relieve their condition or not? All these variables create different manifestations with different possible outcomes. A Bi Syndrome in the knee joint of a twenty-five-year-old yoga student, for example, is different than the same Bi Syndrome in a fifty-year-old retired ballet dancer. Young yoga students, if they are practicing responsive awareness to their body, have the chance to move the obstruction and prevent its recurrence—which will protect their knee ligaments and cartilage as they age. Older ballet dancers likely have practiced ignoring massive amounts of pain and discomfort associated with the obstruction for decades. Because the Qi stagnated for so long, it will take more effort for them to resolve their pain. It's also likely that the time frame for their healing will be longer than for a responsive twenty-five-year-old yoga student.

So you see that the same syndrome can manifest differently as people and circumstances are different.

The role of internal pathogens

Internal pathogens affect the meridian system as well, but they affect the Organs directly. Abdomen, chest, and Organs are internal. Remember that an Organ system includes the meridians associated with the Organ. And that Meridian Massage is a holistic model requiring attention to all aspects of the person.

Why was the meridian susceptible to external pathogens in the first place? Because the Organ was not functioning well. Why was the Organ not functioning well? One likely big reason is that the internal pathogens, the "negative emotions," were stagnating the flow of Qi within the deep, internal meridian system that links the Organs.

The layers and webs of meridians provide us with a logic that explains why we need to clear our internal world of mental and emotional obstructions that limit the functioning of our Organs. The presenting condition might be "just" a stiff neck that is easily cleared up by one massage treatment. But why does the person return each week with this stiff neck? It's likely because of how the internal pathogens reassert themselves in the system.

It is up to clients to decide what they want to do about this. Do they want to delve into the interior causes of this ongoing energetic imbalance that gives rise to the chronic return of the Bi Syndrome affecting their neck? Do they want to make changes in their lifestyle that will support the health of their Organs? Some people are at a point in their life where they are able, willing, and ready to do this work, and others are not.

Likewise, some practitioners are interested in this type of work and some are not. Helping clients discover the deeper changes that need to occur in order to prevent Bi Syndromes from recurring is a more challenging service. Moving from Bi Syndromes to underlying Organ patterns expands your expertise and scope of practice while bringing lasting relief to your clients' suffering. As a practitioner, if you want to support clients with their inner work, you must do yours first and maintain an ongoing practice of inner awareness and growth.

Principles for relieving Bi Syndromes

As mentioned above, Bi Syndromes most often arise along Yang meridians because Yang is more external and exposed to the climatic factors. Your initial intention is to clear the meridians of the pathogens (Heat, Cold, Wind, Damp) in order to relieve the pain. Then you can look into what needs to be done to prevent them from returning. There are five main things to know as you start to clear them.

Essentials for clearing out Bi Syndromes:

1. The actual site of the pain is the location of the blockage (the place where the Wind, Damp, Cold, Heat is lodged in the meridian).

2. Take note of the meridian where the pain is, that is, identify the meridian that needs your help.

3. We always want to keep external pathogens moving in an external rather than internal direction. So, focus on the Yang meridians, bring activity to them, play with the notion of moving the Wind, Cold, Damp, Heat out by opening nearby points, by contacting the whole meridian, and by opening distal points on the fingers and toes to invite the pathogen to leave. This is often described as opening the door and politely encouraging the grumpy guest to leave.

4. Apply the opposite climate factor to the area of blockage. Use heat on cold, cold on heat, dry on damp. With Wind, open the whole meridian so it has a place to move and guide it out by opening local points and distal points.

5. Once the blockage is relieved (the block is the Wind, Cold, Damp, Heat), the Qi will flow and rebalance, which manifests as no more pain.

How to "open" points

I don't have a secret formula for opening or closing points. Many sources advise moving in clockwise or counterclockwise directions to open or close points. This approach never worked for me.

My experience is that allowing for a direct connection of my Qi with the client's Qi creates the guidance for the details of opening a point, for moving blockages, for increasing Qi. Honestly, for any treatment intention I have, I rely on the inherent wisdom of Qi.

I spend a fair amount of my day wondering about Qi, practicing forms of Qi Gong, yoga, breathing, and contemplation in order to develop my ability to feel Qi and be guided by Qi. I have been practicing this for many years. While working with a client, I am often in a kind of meditative state, asking myself to feel Qi, to sense Qi, and allowing my Qi and my hands to answer by contacting the meridians and points. In this state it is as if I am witnessing my work rather than directing it.

As far as I know, the Tao, the Mysterious Source of Nature, is to be followed, not directed. So my feeling is that it is better for me to learn how to be with and respond to the guidance of this Source moment by moment in my sessions, rather than to concern myself with rigid rules about how to open a point. All of my hands-on work is revealed in the moment, in the context of the client's unique situation. As long as I am willing to be guided, my hands will find a way to "open the point."

Preventing Bi Syndromes

To prevent Bi Syndromes, it is important to identify the prevalent climatic factor that invades your client's meridian system. Matching that climatic factor with its associated Element and Organ system gives you big clues about where to direct your future sessions.

For instance, if your client is prone to Wind invading their meridian system, you know that something is out of balance with their Wood Element. By knowing everything associated with the Wood Element, you can support your client to resolve issues related to the Liver and Gallbladder Organs. By asking better questions directed to particular elements, you will have a better sense of the underlying energetic imbalance. Based on what you learn, you can then suggest simple lifestyle adjustments based on the season, flavors, and activities. These lifestyle adjustments will support the work accomplished in the session as well as provide an avenue for lasting change and transformation.

PATHOGEN	SYMPTOMS
Wind	The pain wanders from place to place. "Today my shoulder hurts but yesterday it was my elbow."
Cold	The pain is very severe and localized in one place.
Damp	The pain is severe but not as bad as Cold. Also local with swelling.
Heat	The pain is acute, hot, red, and local.

" In the old days the sages treated disease by preventing illness before it began, just as a good government or emperor was able to take the necessary steps to avert war. Treating an illness after it has begun is like suppressing revolt after it has broken out. If someone digs a well when thirsty or forges weapons after becoming engaged in battle, one cannot help but ask: Are not these actions too late?" [29]

3: Abdominal Massage

The most direct way to affect the Organ systems is to massage the organs. Using touch, breath, awareness, and communication, client and practitioner work together to awaken the resources of each Organ system and Element. We utilize associated meridians and points to support the flow of Qi through the entire web of an Organ system. This chapter addresses how Meridian Massage approaches the process.

This kind of abdominal massage is very specific. It is a combined endeavor of practitioner and client. The practitioner has to understand all the "ingredients" of the abdomen, the location of the organs, and the locations of meridians and points. He or she also must have the ability to be present, centered, and available for the client. Only practitioners who have taken the time to investigate their own abdomen and Organs, meridians, Qi, Life Force, body-mind-spirit are really capable of offering this work to others.

Overview and Context

Organ systems are webs made of physical, emotional, mental, and spiritual threads. By contacting the physical organs in the abdomen, we contact the center of the web. The potential for this type of massage is that we can have a fuller experience of our lives.

Imbalance or dis-ease arises from disunity and imbalance of the Organs. There is no separation between the Elements, the Organs, Yin, Yang, and Qi. The various manifestations that we can name ultimately arise from the One, the Mysterious Source of Nature. The physical reference or location of that undifferentiated Qi within a human is in our form, our body-mind-spirit.

The Qi now flowing in our meridians was absorbed, transformed, and made available to us by our Organs. We work our way inward, towards the One, by working with the Organs and meridians and points. When we commune with the Organs in this way, all the separate "labels" of Yin, Yang, Elements, and Organs disappear. Eventually, we are able to commune with our "center" and know our individual Life-Force as a ray emanating from the Mysterious Source of Nature.

This claim may sound exaggerated—beyond the possibilities of simple abdominal massage. But when we consider the many layers of physical, emotional, mental, and spiritual threads contained within the abdomen we see the potential.

Our modern, Westernized culture tends to value the intellect, the brain, the linear, the categorization of life within the confines of what can be measured, "objectively known" and proven in keeping with scientific method. This direction has led many people away from their gut instincts, their abdomen, their felt senses, emotions, intuition, and connection with their own Life-Force.

As individuals, we may notice over time that it is difficult to feel our abdominal area, the motion of our diaphragm, the ebb and flow of our emotions and intuitions. All of this can be reclaimed when we bring our awareness to our abdomen, and more precisely to the organs and breath. When we return with awareness, curiosity, and support to the Organs, all of the associations of the Elements are there, ready to be re-awakened. Our Organs literally provide us not only with physical nutrients, but with the wisdom of the Elements of Nature. This is why I make such a lofty claim of abdominal massage.

Going in this direction is going in the opposite direction of Western society and enculturation. It takes perseverance, courage, and good company. The reward, though, is access to the whole range of human potential—not just the portion that lives in the brain, in the intellect. When we are able to access the wisdom of our abdomen and the resources of all of our organs, we are more fully equipped to live a life of fuller expression.

Foundational Ideas

- The abdomen is a sacred place, it is our Center.

- Qi is essential to life. Qi is our Life-Force.

- The organs are part of a larger, energetic web known as an Organ system. The Organ system is understood to include the physical organ. For example, the Liver Organ system includes the physical liver as well as the Liver Meridian, Spring, Wind, Tendons, Ligaments, Shouting, Anger, Kindness, Assertion, the color Green, the Sour Taste, Eyes.

- Organs absorb, transform, store, and move Qi.

- Massaging the abdomen is a way to open the flow of Qi between the Organs. When the Qi in the abdomen is flowing smoothly, the Organs receive the nutrition and information they require to support our life to the fullest.

- Stuck or blocked (stagnant) Qi results in pain, cramps, gas, acid reflux, constipation, spastic colon, gall stones, sluggish liver, and more.

- Every Organ has an emotion associated with it. When the Qi of this Organ is stuck, that emotion is stuck also. As we move the Qi of the Organ, the emotion begins to flow also, which accounts for the expression of emotion often experienced during abdominal massage.

- Qi has a native intelligence and an inherent ability to balance and harmonize. Once the Qi is supported to move, it will re-establish harmony and balance. The massage therapist's job is to support the motion of Qi, always knowing that the Qi will guide the work.

Qi has a wisdom of its own. When working with another person, Qi, or the mysterious Force of the Universe, is the most important ingredient to the session. This Force cannot be fooled, and, equally, it will guide the willing practitioner through the session. But to know how to commune with this Force, one must find it in themselves first. Where is it? Most definitely it is accessed from within the abdomen, in the center.

Five Elements and Abdominal Massage

Each organ in the abdomen corresponds to one of the Elements. By contacting an Organ, we contact the Element. Here is a list of Organs that can be contacted in the abdomen and their associated Elements.

ORGAN	ELEMENT
Stomach	Earth
Pancreas	Earth
Small Intestine	Fire
Large Intestine	Metal
Liver	Wood
Gallbladder	Wood
Bladder	Water

Important Points to Consider about the Abdomen

- It was in the abdomen of our biological Mother that we came into physical form.

- Our navel was our first source of nourishment—our literal lifeline.

- The enteric nervous system, a system of nerves as large as the spinal cord, wraps around the gastrointestinal tract. This "private nervous system" of the intestines utilizes the same neuro-transmitters as are found in the brain.

- The enteric nervous system is often referred to as the "the second brain."

- Organs in the abdomen digest the food and liquids we eat and are vital to sustaining our life.

- The abdomen has no bones to protect it.

- Below the lower border of the abdomen, the pelvic area holds the internal and external reproductive organs.

- We habitually store or stuff emotions in the abdomen.

- The abdomen is at the physical center of a human body.

- Breath and the abdomen are intimately connected. The diaphragm separates the thoracic cavity (which holds the heart and lungs) and the abdominal cavity. Movement of the diaphragm as we breathe changes the shape of the abdominal cavity, massages the organs, and creates movement.

- Although we do not massage the lungs and heart directly, creating space in the abdomen for the motion of the diaphragm directly affects the amount of space these vital organs have.

Elaborations:

The abdomen has no bones. Whereas the thoracic cavity is protected by the rib cage, the abdomen lacks the physical protection of bones. Energetically, we don't share this area casually. We protect and guard it in "invisible" ways. Many people for example hold their muscles tightly across the abdomen, even overdeveloping the abdominal muscles. When the abdominal muscles are held too tightly, the motion of the diaphragm is restricted, which restricts the space of the thoracic cavity and the depth of the breath.

We habitually store or stuff emotions in the abdomen. Physiologically, the intestines have the function of sorting nutrients (what we need) from waste (what we don't need and can't use). The intestines sort, absorb what we need, and move the excess along. The large intestine and rectum have the function of letting go, of excreting what is not necessary.

These physiological functions are mirrored energetically by the ingesting, sorting, remembering, and letting go of the events of our life. A large amount of emotional information is stored in the abdomen. When we bring our attention to the abdomen, we are bringing awareness to all of the events of our life, many of which we have forgotten, but remain stored there unconsciously.

The abdomen is at the physical center of a human body. There's a lot of talk about and direction to "connect with our center." Many Eastern cultures value being "centered" as an inward state of stability that allows for flexible, responsive, wise interaction with the world around us and within us. Where is our "center," and what is it? Though it is not much of a consideration in Western philosophy or medicine, most traditional cultures refer to it. It is a constant presence in Taoism, the philosophical basis of Classical Chinese medicine.

Thinking of our "center of gravity" is one way to locate our center. It is a location, a site of energy, a center of balance, a place of connection between "me" and the Mysterious Source of Nature to which I am intricately connected whether I am aware of it or not. It is a place within the abdomen that we must find for ourselves and that we must come to understand solely through our individual experience of being with it, of being connected.

Guidelines for Abdominal Massage

1. Safety. The client must feel safe. Safety is encouraged when the massage therapist:

- Feels grounded, centered, and present.
- Is confident, fluid, and precise with draping.
- Is confident, fluid, and precise when locating anatomical landmarks.
- Follows the exhale when increasing pressure, slows or releases pressure on the inhale.

2. Abdominal Breathing:

- The movement of the breath naturally massages the organs.
- Breath brings awareness to the abdomen.
- Abdominal breathing brings the most air and Qi into the lungs.
- Generally, we can all use a little coaching to support abdominal breathing.

3. Patience:

- Emotions are stored in the abdominal organs. In general, people "store" emotions in the organs to be "dealt with" at a later date. Commonly, this date is put off until we forget that we even stored emotions there at all. As you bring your client's awareness to the abdomen, to their organs, these emotions may want to come to the surface, to move, to release, to be "dealt with."

- Your client may feel very vulnerable as these emotions come back to their consciousness. Now they have a "choice" to make, to recognize and feel what is coming up, or to move away (defend) from the emotions. This can be very confusing and/or frightening, and the client may feel vulnerable. For these reasons the massage therapist must practice patience, presence, and kindness.

- Using associated meridians and points, the massage therapist can help dissipate the intensity of emotions or sensations that are arising within a certain Organ.

4. Movement, Space, Responsiveness:

- Healthy organs move (peristalsis), live in a fluid environment, and are massaged by the motion of the diaphragm as it moves up and down as we breathe in and out. Abdominal muscles support the back and help contain the abdomen. Healthy abdominal muscles are responsive and flexible, and allow the motion of abdominal breathing.

- The main intention of abdominal massage is to create space for the organs and diaphragm, to support their motion and the circulation of blood, Qi, and nerve impulses.

Given the multiple physiological, psychological, and spiritual aspects of this area, it can be a challenge to massage the abdomen. The Organ systems of Chinese medicine offer us an anchor when working on the abdomen. Abdominal massage brings all of the theory of the Organs to life.

Touching the Organs, we awaken the Qi. As we work with our client to loosen the protection around the Organs, Qi is released and needs a place to flow. In some cases the flow has been blocked for years or even decades. We massage the meridians and points with the intention of creating space for this unleashed Qi to flow. This energy becomes available to the rest of the web of meridians and can be circulated to other areas of the body that may have been lacking Qi.

Utilizing the meridians and points, we create space for Qi that in many cases has been held out of our conscious experience for years. Sometimes this process includes memories that have been long forgotten, and with that comes a release of emotion. The flowing of emotion mirrors the flowing of Qi. There is no need to "do" anything with emotional expressions beyond holding a quiet, supportive, and sacred space for clients as they experience this movement. Equally as frequent as an emotional expression is a simple deep breath, a sigh, a softening of the brow, a flush of heat or cool, a bubbling up of joy and laughter.

The Qi of each Organ has a direction of energetic flow. For example, Wood is up and out while Metal is down and in. Having knowledge of these directions of energetic flow allows the practitioner to open meridians and points related to the Organ being worked with. As we combine contact with the Organs with thoughtful contact of related meridians and points, we support the unwinding and releasing of stagnant Qi held in the Organs.

Once again, the intention of all of this work is to support the return of flowing Qi to the client's entire body-mind-spirit. The simple recipe of health is that abundant, flowing Qi gives rise to vitality, health, peace, happiness, and the ability to respond more gracefully to the myriad changes and challenges of life.

It is worth repeating that unblocking meridians is a combined effort of client and practitioner. Bringing awareness to the Organs and the sometimes long held "knots" of Qi requires a safe place and a willingness to explore oneself. We support our clients by reminding them to follow the flow of the Qi associated with the Organ system we are contacting. We amplify that movement by contacting meridians and points that support a given direction of Qi flow.

This is a large amount of information to understand and apply. One's own experiential understanding of unblocking Qi flow between Organs and in the meridians of the sacred and private space of the abdomen is a necessary component of being able to offer this work to another.

Practice principles for massaging the abdomen

1. Increase pressure during the client's exhale, lighten pressure during the inhale. Taking the time to match your pressure with the client's breath will result in more trust and better contact with the underlying organs.

2. Establish verbal communication as you apply pressure. Use language to continually invite your client to feel where your pressure is. We do this in order to support them to become more aware of their abdomen. Having a clear sense of the organs, being able to bring awareness and allow for sensation offers the client a practical pathway to the resources of their Organs.

3. Massaging specifically in the abdomen and contacting the Organs releases a great deal of energy, even if there is no noticeable sensation of it by the client. This energy (Qi) needs a place to go, so open the shoulders, hips, and neck to give places for that Qi to flow. Apply pressure to the meridians and points to encourage the opening of the meridians and the flow of Qi. (If you do not "drain" the Qi that gets released during abdominal massage, there is a likelihood that it will only become stagnated and stuck again. This will manifest as a stiff neck, headache, tension, or pain in the limbs or even in the abdominal organs themselves.)

4. Allow for a progression over several sessions rather than to overdo it in a single session. Sometimes a person has a great many unconscious memories and much associated emotion stored in the abdomen. They may be eager to "deal with it" all at once, or the practitioner may urge the client to keep delving into material that is too overwhelming. Massage is medicine, and to be effective it must be given in the right dose.

5. After working in the abdomen, always be sure to open the hips, shoulders, and neck in order to support the flow of Qi in all directions away from the abdomen. As mentioned above, Qi that is released from massaging Organs needs a place to flow; otherwise it will build up at areas of stagnation and possibly cause muscle spasms, cramps, emotional outbursts after the session, insomnia, fatigue, or just a sense of "not feeling good," ungrounded, or anxious.

4: Bringing It All Together

Now that you have the various pieces of the puzzle, how are you to actually "do the work?"

The abdomen is the central starting place. All the theory you have covered is practically expressed in the abdominal organs, because they are the physical reference place for each Organ system. Organ systems entwine with the Five Elements. The Five Elements emerge from Yin and Yang. Yin and Yang emerge from the Mysterious Source of Nature, the One, the Tao.

Regardless of how you begin a session, a good portion of your time should go into contacting organs in the abdomen. Working with these organs is the most direct way to support the flow of Qi within and between them. Working with these organs, we communicate with the many layers of Element, Organ System, Mind, Body, and Spirit all at once.

Abdominal massage, again, is a cooperative process between the practitioner and the client. This cooperation gives the practitioner an opportunity to guide the client into a deeper self-awareness. When a client is consciously present within his or her own energy system, the stage is set for truly unblocking meridians and allowing the Qi to flow and balance. When the Qi is abundant and flowing, the result is harmony and health in Body, Mind, and Spirit.

Once the Qi is awakened and moving in the abdomen, use points on the limbs and head to support the continuing flow of Qi. The points you choose are guided by the indications given in Part 2. By listening carefully to your client's concerns before working with them, you will have a sense of what points and meridians will guide the Qi back to balance.

With practice and experience you will find yourself weaving these principles into each particular situation of your hands-on healing in a new way. Each practitioner will have their own individual expression of Meridian Massage, in keeping with our individuality as people. Likewise, each client will have unique needs.

Working with Qi means being open to surprises, listening to your inner wisdom, connecting with your own Qi in order to gracefully respond to the Qi of others. By contacting the abdominal organs, meridians, and points, you are able to connect directly with Qi–and that opens a world of possibility for you and your client.

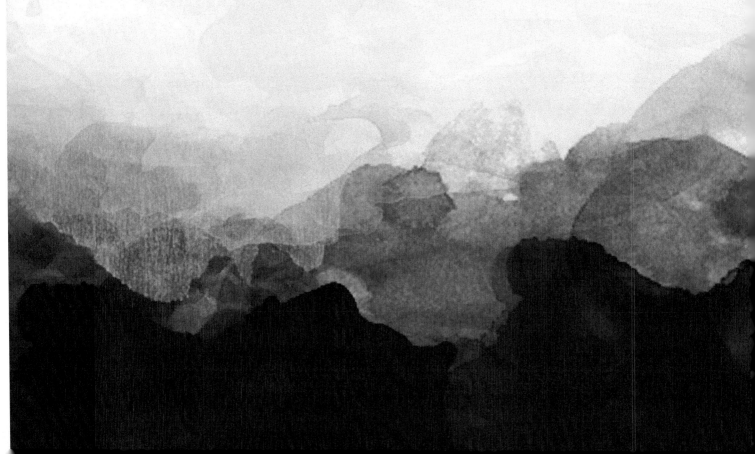

Part 4
_____

Common Conditions:
The Meridian Massage Approach to Common Conditions Encountered in a Hands-on Healing Practice

1: Conditions Alphabetically

This chapter offers guidance for seeing some common conditions through the lens of Meridian Massage. Always keep in mind that you are working with an individual who shows signs of an imbalance, rather than treating an identified condition.

Do not limit yourself to the suggestions given here. The analyses and approaches offered are meant to be starting points for your understanding of these ailments in the context of the Meridian Massage perspective. At times I give point suggestions—again, these are given as starting places rather than rigid treatment regimens.

You will notice that different conditions have similar approaches. This is because certain patterns of imbalance are at the root of many manifestations. For instance, the approach is similar for hyperactivity (ADHD) and insomnia. These two different conditions have a similar root imbalance of too much Fire in relation to Water. This issue highlights a key difference between Classical Chinese medicine (the basis for Meridian Massage) and Western medicine. By knowing the underlying energetic imbalance, we can predict many manifestations that Western medicine would treat as separate and unrelated conditions. Addressing the underlying imbalance not only resolves the cause of the condition, but also prevents the manifestation of seemingly unrelated (from the Western perspective) future conditions.

Please think about these in conjunction with the next chapter, Conditions by Element. The two chapters complement one another. Where this one orders conditions alphabetically, seeing the conditions also by Elements will support your understanding of related manifestations that may spring from a similar imbalance of Qi.

Addiction

Associated Element: Wood
Associated Organ: Liver

Analysis

Addiction affects the Liver, which clears toxins from the Blood. The Liver is always impacted by drugs—legal and illegal, prescribed and over-the-counter—whether the user is addicted or not. The Liver is sensitive to overheating and many drugs add heat into the Organ systems.

When the Liver is overwhelmed by toxins, Qi stagnates and the balance of the Wood Element is disturbed. On a bad day, the Liver can be very cranky, grumpy, and short-tempered. On a really bad day, the Qi stagnation manifests as anger, explosive temper, extreme frustration that blocks one's ability to bring creative inspirations from the Water Element toward manifestation. The feeling of Qi stagnation can be physically painful and emotionally exhausting.

Liver Qi wants to move, grow, and expand. Thwarted, the Liver Qi tends to react, to go into fight-or-flight mode in order to push through obstacles. It doesn't feel good or satisfying to be hemmed in by restrictions. How we respond to not feeling good internally may be to numb the "this doesn't feel good" sensation with substances or behaviors that block the sensation.

As we continue to block that sensation, we might feel good (because we have numbed the "this doesn't feel good" sensations), but we never learn to cope with the sensation we are blocking. Whenever the unwanted sensation begins to arise again, we repeat the behavior that blocks it. After a while, we have ourselves an addiction to the thing or behavior that blocks our internal negative feeling.

The Wood Element is a key player in addiction because it is our protector. On a psychological level, the blocking of the negative feeling is a mechanism of protecting oneself from memories or circumstances that give rise to the negative feelings that we want to block. This is a protective survival mechanism. Wood protects the Life Force held in Water, as well as growing the seeds of our creativity.

We all have our defense mechanisms, our protective mechanisms. Some of these involve substances, some are behaviors, some are thought-patterns or restrictions. They help us maintain a barrier between our sense of ourselves, and circumstances or events that were/are too traumatic for us to cope with consciously.

Approach

Depending on the individual, the addiction, and the extent of physically manifested conditions, the healing approaches and outcomes are varied, as with any other condition of imbalance.

The first step will always be supporting the client to feel the sensation of "this doesn't feel good." As people move toward that sensation, they inevitably encounter their habitual defense system. It is at this point that the practitioner must gracefully step in as a safe, reliable, and trustworthy guide who can help the client dismantle the defenses and face the feelings, memories, and sensations he or she has been avoiding.

What does "stepping in" look like? Invite your client to feel their breath as a way of bringing the attention inward. Make contact with the abdomen and work around the liver area while continuing to coach your client to stay aware of the sensations they encounter in the area of your contact. This process encourages the awareness of what has been hidden or ignored and suppressed in the abdomen. It is likely that they will become aware of something unpleasant and turn away from that sensation, as they habitually do. This can look like them falling asleep, holding their breath, starting an unrelated conversation, contracting the abdominal muscles tightly, staring off into space and taking their attention out of the abdomen, etc. Use the principles covered in the chapter on abdominal massage (Part 3, Chapter 3, pp. 218-225) to support your clients in doing the hard and courageous work of feeling into what has been avoided for so long. Then, use distal points to encourage the Qi that is released in the abdomen to flow—the points LI-4 and LV-3 are particularly good for stimulating Qi flow throughout the meridian network.

Alzheimer's Disease

Associated Element: Water
Associated Organ: Kidney

Analysis

This condition most often affects the brains of older people. That the brain and aging are involved points to the Kidney as the Organ to consider.

The Kidneys store the Essence, our pre-Heaven Qi. This precious resource of Life Force dwindles as we age. As it decreases, our ability to form Qi and Blood also diminishes and in turn affects all our Organ systems and functions.

The tissue of the Kidneys is the bones and the marrow inside the bones. In Chinese medicine, the brain, spinal cord, and bone marrow all fill the spaces within bones. This shows us a direct connection between the Kidneys and the brain.

Approach

The condition we call Alzheimer's Disease is based on a deficiency of Kidney Essence. We can't replace the Kidney Essence, but we can conserve what is left. Conserving the Essence relies on getting good post-Heaven Qi, enough rest, and relaxation. See the sections on the Spleen and the Kidneys in Part 1, Chapter 4: Organ Systems for more details about this process (pp. 68-70 and pp. 76-78).

To consolidate the Kidney Essence, use KD-3. To nourish Kidney Yin in particular use KD-6. The Du extraordinary vessel is associated with the brain. Massage the Du vessel on the head and focus on the point DU-20 at the top of the head to stimulate the brain. Use the Master Point combination of SI-3 and BL-62 to further stimulate the Du and enliven the brain.

Asthma

Associated Element: Metal
Associated Organs: Lung, Large Intestine

Analysis

Any issue related to the respiratory system is part of the Lung Organ system and involves the Metal Element.

The Lung Organ system is the Yin Organ of the Metal Element. It includes the nose, nasal passages, trachea, lung organs, skin, the color white, the season of Fall, and the emotions of grief and courage. We meet our clients at a moment in time. If in that moment they are suffering from asthma, we must remember that this asthma is a manifestation at this point in time of an underlying system of Qi. Because the concern is about breathing, we know for sure that the Lung Organ system is involved.

Approach

The relevance of knowing all the associations with the Elements and Organ systems is clear when considering a Western diagnosis such as asthma. Ask questions about the Metal Element, find out about any losses that may be lingering, how is their breathing? Do they have "room to breathe" in their key relationships, within themselves? For what endeavor must they be gathering their courage? Are they able to feel their breath?

Because the Lung is Yin, also explore Yin associations such as nurturing, rest, inner stillness, intuition, receiving, receptivity, mothering.

For many people, feeling the breath and lungs is a foreign idea and a challenging task. The skin gives us boundaries and the sensations of feeling the environment around us. When imbalances arise in the Lung Organ system, our work is to help the person bring his/her attention inward (the season of Fall), feel their breath, feel their lungs, feel themselves, and feel whatever it is emotionally that needs to be felt. We are supporting them to feel the environment within themselves.

This work requires time, space, quiet, compassion, patience, safety, and the guidance of a person who is fully present and peaceful. Through our own practice of going inward and feeling ourselves, we gain the confidence to help others do it.

The main principle here is that each of us knows what is best for ourselves. But getting to that knowing is an adventure that sometimes feels overwhelming, which is why we sometimes need the help of others. The "help" we as practitioners offer our clients through Meridian Massage is guidance back to their connection with themselves, with their Spirit, with their Qi.

"Breath" is a word often used as a translation of Qi. Breath is essential to life. Breath creates movement in the whole body, especially in the chest and abdomen. It infuses the system with fresh Qi and relieves it of used Qi. Coach your clients gently to feel their breath, their lungs, diaphragm, ribs, and the movement of their body in response to the breath. The point of all of this is to help them feel themselves, to open to their own inner voice, and to generate the solutions to their "asthma."

For easy, deep breathing to occur, the abdomen must be relaxed and pliable. Abdominal massage is a key method of opening the breath, as it serves to relax and open the organs. The Large Intestine, the Yang partner of the Lungs, is an important organ to focus on for these respiratory issues.

Letting go is related to the Large Intestine in terms of moving what needs excretion out of the body. Grief and loss involve letting go—often of people, things, or relationships that we were not "ready" to let go of. Attending to the Large Intestine supports the emotional aspect of the Metal Element, it creates space in the abdomen for breathing, and it supports the energetic balance of the Metal Organs—the Lung and Large Intestine.

ADHD (Attention Deficit Hyperactivity Disorder)

Associated Element: Fire
Associated Organ: Heart

Analysis

When the mind is hyperactive and wandering, it is not grounded in the Yin. We look to the Heart and the Fire Element.

Hyperactivity is in the realm of excess of Fire, excess Yang. We see a continuum of excess Fire conditions as we look at insomnia, anxiety, ADHD, high blood pressure, etc. The underlying pattern of this energy gives rise to any number of manifestations. Rather than chasing manifestations, we work toward harmony between Yin and Yang and the Five Elements, and to restore the smooth flow of abundant Qi throughout the meridian system.

Western culture celebrates extroversion, ambition, activity, doing, rising to the top, speed, external credentials, overwork, excessive eating, drinking, sex, talking, thinking, partying, socializing, shopping, accumulation. All things Yang are strongly encouraged, validated, celebrated. There is nothing wrong with loving Yang! Just don't forget about Yin. If you forget about Yin, you will be reminded sooner or later, with manifestations of trouble in your body, mind, relationships, family, career.

At some time the massive excess of Yang will no longer be able to be buoyed by Yin. The Yin will be diminished as it pours itself out to fuel Yang. When the balance tips over an unforeseen and unknown threshold, symptoms will appear.

One gift of knowing about the flow and cycles of Yin and Yang is that we can temper and balance their energies before they get so far out of balance that the manifestations are beyond our ability to survive. This is a tall order for people who live in countries whose cultures have moved to the extreme of Yang. It is challenging for individuals to turn against the tide of culture and society, but not impossible.

Approach

One approach to dealing with this condition is to take the perspective that our inner attention and self-reflection are deficient. By utilizing the inward movement of the Metal Element and the deep quiet of the Water Element, we can balance Fire and Water, Yin and Yang. When the underlying Qi is balanced and flowing, the manifestation is also balanced and flowing.

To balance Fire and Water the point combination of KD-3 and HT-7 is helpful, and also REN-17 combined with REN-6. Suggest lifestyle adjustments based on your knowledge of Fire, Water, and the particulars of your client. When the Fire is consistently excessive compared to Water, we need to let off the extra heat from Fire and increase and consolidate the Water. A gentle walk is a great way to let off heat without exhausting the Kidneys. Taking a short nap in the afternoon restores the Kidney/Water energy.

Anxiety

Associated Element: Fire
Associated Organ: Heart

Analysis

As this condition is an issue of the Shen—Spirit—we are directed to the Heart. The Spirit or Shen resides in the Heart. When the Heart is weak or the Fire Element is excessive, the Spirit has no calm place to reside. The manifestation of this restless Spirit can be anxiety, insomnia, rage, or psychiatric conditions such as schizophrenia.

When Fire blazes out of control it burns things. Think of people getting delusional when they have a very high fever—this is extreme excessive heat. When excessive heat is a chronic condition, it can result in more extreme mental-emotional issues.

Anxiety has our mind in a revved-up state, the whole body and our senses are in a state of vigilant alert for some type of disaster or threat. This is hyper Yang, too much Fire and not enough Water to bring the Fire down. This type of pattern continues itself as the Fire burns off the Blood and Yin, exacerbating the problem.

Approach

Coming back to a fundamental Yin-Yang balance is the path back to a centered, composed, quiet mind. In the midst of anxiety, the attention is very much directed outward and often to future events. This is a type of extroversion, a form of outward-directed attention that neglects the inner world. Yang, Fire, extroversion is balanced with Yin, Water, introversion. Turning the attention inward and to the present moment can be very challenging for a person caught up in excess Fire and anxiety, but it is necessary.

Attending to the breath, feeling the breath, the lungs, the movement of the body in response to the breath are all ways to open the path for awareness to turn inward and balance the Yang extroversion.

In the center is the seat of individual wisdom and knowing. This is precisely the remedy for the anxiety, so support your clients to turn toward themselves and feel their own center.

For specific points and lifestyle adjustments to balance Yin and Yang, see ADHD above.

Arthritis

Associated Element: Water
Associated Organ: Kidneys

Analysis

Muscle and joint pain fall into the category of what we call Bi Syndromes. "Bi" here means "obstruction," and these kinds of pain arise from obstructions in the meridians. The Qi in the meridians is obstructed and gathers at a specific site. As the Qi gathers in that place, it creates pressure, distention, pain, cramping in the local area. See the chapter on Bi Syndromes for more detail (Part 3, Chapter 2 p.211).

Depending on what causes the obstruction, there are different types of pain. The four main pathogens are Wind, Cold, Damp, and Heat, but Heat is not as common as the other three.

Depending on the main pathogen there are different symptoms (refer to p.213).

These are literal pathogens. "My pain is worse when it is damp and cold" is real. When someone tells you this, you are being given a huge clue about the main pathogens involved.

Approach

In practice, Wind, Damp, and Cold often enter together and it really doesn't matter which came first. The treatment is to open the obstruction, to move the Qi. When you know that Cold and Damp are involved, this is the time to add dry heat to your treatment. Moxibustion (a traditional heat application using dried mugwort) is the classic treatment for Cold, Damp Bi Syndromes.

Wind enters meridians when they are empty. Imagine an empty hall. When the door opens, the Wind rushes in. In contrast, when the meridians are full of flowing Qi, the Wind cannot enter. So the short-term treatment is to move the obstruction, and the prevention is to keep the meridians full of flowing Qi.

When the arthritis is severe and chronic, keep the person out of the weather conditions that cause the symptoms to flare up. Stay out of the Wind, Damp, and Cold, or at least bundle up! In the West we often think that climate factors are "old wives tales." In this case and many others, the old wives knew what they were talking about!

Arthritis affects the bones, so factor in the Kidneys. Notice that the climatic factor that is associated with the Kidneys is Cold (Winter). Too much Cold injures the Kidneys. Add in points to nourish the Kidneys, such as KD-3 and BL-23. (See also Part 3, Chapter 2, Obstruction Syndromes—Bi Syndromes.)

Carpal Tunnel Syndrome

Associated Element: Wood
Associated Organ: Liver

Analysis

Pain syndromes of the muscles, tendons, and joints most often result from blockages in the meridian that prevent the flow of Qi—the obstruction syndromes or Bi Syndromes mentioned above and in Part 3, Chapter 2. The longer the obstruction has been present, the more difficult it is to remove (but not impossible).

Carpal tunnel is often the result of a long-term obstruction and a long period of overuse. Obstructions affect Qi first. If the Qi is obstructed for a long time, Blood begins to stagnate also, and the pain increases. Blood is material and thicker than Qi, so the resolution takes longer, requires more effort and consistent attention. The local structures have become stiff and non-functional during the time their supply of Qi and Blood circulation have been reduced, depriving them of energy and nourishment.

Stagnation can build up anywhere in the body. When it occurs at the wrist, Western medicine defines it as carpal tunnel syndrome; we refer to it as severe Qi and Blood stagnation.

Approach

This condition is another type of overuse syndrome. As with most overuse syndromes, part of what causes it is ignoring body signals such as pain, discomfort from postures required to perform an action, and the need for a break. Addressing this pattern of behavior is an essential part of preventing recurrence and further injury.

There are six meridians crossing the wrist, three anterior (Heart, Pericardium, Lung) and three posterior (Small Intestine, San Jiao, Large Intestine). Examine each meridian. Ask your clients to trace their pain along their arm, wrist, and hand to help identify which meridian(s) are involved. Locally, the intention is to unblock the meridians and move the Qi and Blood.

The Liver is responsible for keeping the meridians open in order to ensure the smooth flow of Qi. The tissue of the Wood Element is the tendons and ligaments. These factors point us to the Liver and the Gallbladder meridians and points to support the underlying flow of Qi in the meridians in order to both relieve and prevent carpal tunnel syndrome (as well as any other overuse syndromes).

Depression

Associated Elements: Metal, Fire, Water
Associated Organs: Lung, Heart, Kidneys

Analysis

Yang brings light, movement, extroversion, communication, passion, and joy to Yin's dark, still, quiet, reflective, content, creative center. When they are in balance and harmony, we pass through our relative ups and downs with ease in the course of a basically happy and content life.

The energy of depression is down, "depressed," and gravitating inward, unrelating, dull, fading, limp, inertial. What we see in this condition is a lack of Yang. It may also be that the Yang is so restricted that it cannot express itself—the person is unable to contact it.

Every Organ is associated with an emotion. This notion is not just a concept or a metaphor, it is a reality. Notice how you express and feel joy, happiness, and love—it comes right out of your heart center. If that expression is unavailable or unable to flow, you may feel depressed.

Fire and Water must be in balance as two poles of constancy that ground the entire being. Being out of balance results in chaos through the whole system, making it hard to predict where or how this imbalance will manifest. One way is depression. The Fire sinks into the Water, becoming extinguished or so contained that it cannot rise.

The Metal Element gives us the ability to feel ourselves. Metal also gives us the courage to face our situations and work our way out of difficulty. Often there is a lack of feeling and a sense of isolation during depression, which clues us in to the connection of the Metal Element with this condition.

Approach

There are many Elements at play with depression, yet there are few general guidelines to consider.

One: Support people to feel themselves. People are depressed for many reasons, facing those circumstances can be overwhelming. Be aware of the tremendous amount of energy and courage it takes for your clients to feel what is actually going on within themselves.

Two: Support the connection to the Heart. We do this in order to reconnect our clients with their source of Yang, love, fire, compassion, expression. Fire can soften the cold isolation of out-of-balance Metal.

Three: Support the balance and connection of Yin and Yang. The communication and harmony of Yin and Yang are essential in order for people to have full expression of themselves. With extreme conditions such as depression, it is a good guess that Yin and Yang are not communicating. That disconnect can manifest in many ways. Depression is one. Hyperactivity is another.

To balance Yin and Yang, work to bring a felt sense of connection between the heart (Fire area) and the lower abdomen (Water area). Use REN-17 combined with REN-6, BL-15 combined with BL-23, and HT-7 combined with KD-3 to support that connection. To nourish the Metal Element use LU-1, LU-2, and LU-7.

Fibromyalgia

Associated Elements: Earth, Wood
Associated Organs: Spleen, Liver

Analysis

Muscles are the tissue of the Earth Element. Chronic pain throughout the muscle system points to the Earth Element and the Wood Element. The Wood Element is responsible for the smooth flow of Qi throughout the meridian system. Pain that wanders is due to Wind. Wind is the climatic factor of the Wood Element. Blockages in meridians stagnate Qi and the result is pain. Meridian blockages show in various areas in this condition, which accounts for the sensations of pain in various areas associated with fibromyalgia.

Approach

In general, we want to nourish the Earth Element and soothe the Wood Element. Consider the associations of the Earth Element and ask your client questions about their sense of safety, satisfaction, nourishment, mothering, etc. Learn about the dynamic of Wood and Earth within this particular person by asking about their ambitions, how they handle anger and frustration, where they want to expand, etc.

To nourish the Earth Element, use SP-6 combined with ST-36, ST-36 combined with ST-25, and abdominal massage. Support the Earth by encouraging the client to literally connect more with the Earth by being in Nature, working in a garden, lying on the ground, feeling their feet on the ground, preparing their own nutritious food, etc.

To soothe the Wood Element use LV-3, the entire Gallbladder meridian, and main points such as GB-20, GB-21, GB-30, GB-34, GB-41. Use caution when applying pressure to any points, especially the Gallbladder points as clients are often ultra-sensitive. Use only a few points in the first session so that the client can experience the work in a small dose and ensure that it does not create a flare-up.

Frozen Shoulder

Associated Element: Wood
Associated Organ: Liver

Analysis

The tissue of the Wood Element is the sinews, the tendons, the ligaments, and the fibrous connective tissues. Frozen shoulder points to restriction, stagnation, and dryness in the Wood Element.

Approach

In addition to looking for problems affecting or associated with the Wood Element, examine the individual meridians that travel across the shoulder (Large Intestine, San Jiao, Small Intestine, Lung, Pericardium, Heart). Palpate along the meridians to pinpoint which ones are most tender to your client. This will give you additional information to work with.

SI-9 and SI-10 are particularly effective for shoulder conditions. LU-1 and LU-2 may also be good points to use for local movement of Qi.

All of the meridians found on the hand cross the shoulder at various locations. The Gallbladder meridian (see diagram on p. 138) may also be involved as it traverses the side of the body; it is always involved in one-sided (meaning manifested only on one side) conditions, and is part of the Wood Element. GB-20 and GB-21 can be utilized to create local movement of Qi in the neck and shoulder. GB-34 is the Influential Point for tendons and ligaments and should always be used in this circumstance.

Herniated Disc

Associated Element: Water
Associated Organs: Kidney, Bladder

Analysis

Bones, discs, marrow, the brain, and the spinal cord are in the realm of the Water Element. Disc bulge, herniation, and degeneration are issues related to the Kidney. Note also that the Bladder meridian (see diagram on p. 116) runs parallel along the entire vertebral column and the kidneys themselves are located at the lower back.

Herniated discs are often the result over time of overuse, excess straining of the spine, or lack of sufficient motion. Why do we overuse our bodies? What happened to working hard, taking a rest, pausing now and then, and getting help with the heavy lifting? What happened to responding to our desire to get up from our desks and move? We repair, regenerate, restore our physical structure while we sleep and rest. Too much work (excess Yang) and not enough rest (Yin) will one day result in damage to some structures.

Yin is the nourishing basis for Yang. Yang is what is seen; it gives us motion, activity, "doing." But all this activity is fueled by Yin. We see a tree but not its roots. The health of the tree is entirely dependent on its roots and the soil that holds the roots.

How do we nourish our roots? We nourish and consolidate our Kidney Yin, the Essence. It is simple: eat when you are hungry, sleep when you are tired, follow your heart.

Practicing simplicity is a challenge, yet a necessity for a long, happy, healthy life.

Ignoring the body's signals, pushing through pain and fatigue, sets us up for injury. Disc injuries are often the result of not listening and overworking. These actions are in direct opposition to the wisdom of Yin that encourages us to listen inwardly, to soften, to yield, to be. The quality of the Yin-Yang balance within every person is different. In order for Yin and Yang to truly balance, they must cooperate.

In order for them to cooperate, we must listen inwardly to ourselves, to each of our Organs, and adjust our behaviors and activities according to what we hear. We are changing all the time—in relation to the seasons, the time of day, the cycles of the Universe "outside of" us, and the cycle of our own individual lifetime. Taking time for ourselves is not just a self-indulgent luxury, it is a necessity.

Unfortunately, many of us only realize the necessity of listening to and responding to the signals our bodies are sending when a chronic condition becomes quite debilitating, as is the case with intervertebral disc issues.

Approach

The best approach is prevention. Coaching and supporting your clients to become more self-aware and responsive to pain signals will go a long way in preventing chronic conditions such as herniated discs. If a person does have a herniation, we can support their healing with meridians, points, and encouragement to listen to and respond to their pain.

Point suggestions: KD-3 and BL-23 to nourish the Kidneys. SI-3 combined with BL-62 is a Master Point combination for the back. Utilize local Bladder points to encourage the flow of Qi in the area of the herniation (gentle or even no pressure depending on the person's situation).

Insomnia

Associated Element: Fire
Associated Organ: Heart

Analysis

At night when Yin overtakes Yang, the Mind rests in the Blood and we sleep. If we can't sleep, that is a sign that Yin is not strong enough to overtake the Yang.

When Yin is diminished, the Blood (Yin) is also diminished. When the Blood is diminished, the Mind (Yang) has no place to rest at night and so it wanders (or spins, creating fantasies of worry, doubt, fear, anger, etc.).

The Heart governs the Blood. The Heart is the residence of the Spirit. Insomnia points us to the Heart. When the Fire is too big for the Water to balance, Yin does not overtake Yang at night, and Yang remains active.

The Mind and Blood are a Yang and Yin pair. Mind is Yang and requires the grounding, gravitational force of Yin Blood to keep it settled and embodied. A restless, busy, sleepless Mind is a sign of imbalance in this pair.

Approach

The Yin Blood needs to be nourished. How do we nourish Yin? Quiet, rest, introspection, being rather than doing, wondering rather than figuring out, eating nourishing food in a relaxing environment, feeling our breath.

Helpful points for hands-on massage work:

P-6 + REN-17 is a beautiful combination for calming the heart and Spirt.

SP-4 + P-6 is a Master Point combination for nourishing the interior, Yin, Blood.
To balance Yin and Yang in general, use KD-3 + HT-7, BL-23 + BL-15, REN-17 + REN-6.

Irritable Bowel Syndrome (IBS)

Associated Element: Metal
Associated Organ: Large Intestine

Analysis

Irritable bowel syndrome affects the Large Intestine. The Large Intestine is the Yang Organ of the Metal Element. Because IBS affects the Large Intestine, we know there must something out of balance with the Metal Element.

Approach

Working from the energetic perspective, notice that we address the same set of issues—loss, grief, letting go, skin, feeling, courage, Fall, white—to "treat" two very different manifestations—IBS and asthma. By addressing the underlying Qi, we can resolve and prevent many different types of manifestations with a relatively simple approach.

Explore the Metal Element associations in order to understand the particular manifestation of IBS. Explore the Yang associations of ambition, expansion, expression, aggression, assertion, anger, and joy, and see how these emotions affect the Large Intestine.

As noted in the next chapter's "Metal" section, the Metal Element is generally neglected in Western cultures. For a longer discussion of the Wood–Metal imbalance, please refer to p. 258 there.

Abdominal massage is key to relieving IBS. We can increase the circulation of Qi and Blood directly to the large intestine with gentle, pain-free massage. Recall from previous discussions that blocking our emotions will block the flow of Qi in meridians. Qi that cannot flow backs up and causes pain, from minor to serious. Additionally, the abdominal organs commonly "store" pent-up emotions. Over time, these stored emotions and emotional blocks can cause damage to the organs.

Working gently in the abdomen and helping your clients meet themselves and the challenging emotions, memories, and beliefs they have stored away can be a great benefit in relieving IBS.

Adding ST-36 combined with ST-25 and SP-15 to abdominal massage is an effective approach to relieving intestinal pain and supporting intestinal health. ST-44, LI-11, and SJ-5 all relieve heat and should be considered during acute flare-ups.

Joint Issues (Joint pain, joint degeneration, arthritis, joint replacements)

Associated Element: Water
Associated Organ: Kidney

Analysis

All conditions of the bones point our attention to the Kidney Organ and the Water Element. Bones are the tissue associated with Water.

As mentioned above for arthritis and for carpal tunnel syndrome, pain syndromes of the muscles, tendons, and joints most often result from blockages in a meridian that prevent the flow of Qi—the obstruction syndromes or Bi syndromes mentioned above and in Part 3, Chapter 2. The longer the obstruction has been present, the more difficult it is to remove (but not impossible). Joint conditions vary in magnitude from a little ache once in a while to chronic pain from the wearing-away of all cartilage that requires replacement or fusion. Regardless of the manifestation, the underlying pattern of blocked flow in the meridian was the original cause (unless the cause was external physical trauma, such as a car accident). Even if physical trauma initiated the condition, the trauma creates local obstruction and stagnation.

What else causes stagnation in the meridians? The external pathogens of Wind, Cold, and Damp are the main causes. Heat is also a cause, although not as common as the other three. Internal pathogens such as fear, anger, worry, grief, sadness, anxiety. Lifestyle choices such as eating foods of poor quality, lack of exercise, lack of recreation, too much work and not enough rest, overeating, over-medicating, and the rest of those "bad habits" we can all recite.

Our bodies send us signals all the time about what they need—signals of thirst, hunger, sleepiness, pain, excitement, cold, hot, enthusiasm, yes, no. The idea is that if we could pay attention to these messages, we would make the little adjustments along the way that would support our well-being. But we learn from family, society, and culture to override these messages.

There is an invisible energetic ability in each of us that allows us to suppress or override the calls of our body. This is a handy and important mechanism for situations where our survival depends on doing that. However, it is often so overused that the pattern of suppression becomes unconscious and seems "normal" to us. This suppressive mechanism blocks the flow of Qi.

If someone makes you very angry, your Qi rises and readies you for a fight. Your muscles infuse with adrenaline, your face might turn red. We all know this sensation, and we all know how to control it. We can contain this upward blast of energy, keep ourselves quiet, contained, polite, and maybe even smile at the person who is triggering us. That ability in appropriate circumstances can save your life and keep you out of trouble. But overused, it blocks the flow of Qi in your Organ systems and meridians. Depending on where the blockage is located, different symptoms arise and grow into bigger, badder symptoms and manifestations.

Approach

Joint issues have something to do with the Water Element, which has many "pieces" to it. So the answer for how to deal with the issue is not always straightforward. But if you keep in mind the range of possibilities and the specific individual who has the symptoms, you can unwind the obstructions and get the Qi flowing again. Depending on the extent of physical manifestation and the lifestyle changes the person is able to make, different expressions of healing can manifest.

Use local points to relieve pain in the affected joints, and then think more broadly about the underlying root cause. Is it from overuse, under use (lack of motion)? Overuse conditions often have a component of pushing through pain rather than responding to pain—how can you support your client to become more sensitive and then make adjustments to reduce wear and tear? Under use conditions often include a component of inertia or aversion to moving. How can you support your clients to be more sensitive to pain caused by lack of motion and help them find healthy movement that they can sustain?

Migraine

Associated Element: Wood
Associated Organ: Liver

Analysis

This condition manifests as acute, extremely painful headache, often located behind one eye, or on one side. Some migraines include visual disturbances as well (ocular migraine).

One-sided manifestations and the eyes call our attention to the Wood Element. Wood energy is strong and moves up and out, just as a tough little weed breaks through hard pavement.

The internal pathway of the Liver meridian goes up the neck and through the head, to the center of the top of the head. Imagine Spring bursting forth in just one day, contained within the small space of your head. Migraine!

Spring is the time of young Yang, which is a very forceful Yang. The Yang aspect of the Wood Element must be balanced with the Yin aspect of the Wood Element. The Yin Organ and the Yang Organ in each Element are what maintain the Yin-Yang balance of that Element—this is true within every Element. So here, even though the Liver is a Yin Organ, it is associated with this young Yang, bursting energy.

Approach

Liver Yang has to be held down by Liver Yin. If the Liver Yin is too weak, the Liver Yang breaks free and blows upward. Wind is the climate associated with Wood. Like an internal tornado, this Wind travels upward. If it goes to the head, it can manifest as a migraine or even a stroke.

The immediate treatment is to release this energy out of the skull and bring it back down. Using meridians and points that direct the Qi down, we can be relatively successful in the moment. Use DU-20 and GB-21 as places to "let the steam off." I think of opening these points to allow the excess Wind out of the head and shoulders as taking the lid off a hot pot. The intention is to give the excess Liver Yang a place to exit through these points rather than getting bound up in the head.

GB-21 will also help move the Qi down. I use the Gallbladder and Bladder meridians along with the points GB-30, GB-34, GB-41, GB-44, and BL-60 to encourage the Qi to move downwards.

Once the immediate crisis is resolved, the client needs to make lifestyle changes and do inner work to nourish the Liver Yin and the Yin of the body in general. By increasing the Yin we create a strong anchor for Yang and keep it from flaring upwards.

Muscle Spasm

Associated Element: Earth
Associated Organ: Spleen

Analysis

Muscle spasms result from Bi Syndromes blocking the meridian so Qi cannot flow. The varying degrees of muscle tension, from "just a little tight" to spasm reflect the degree and duration of the obstruction. Refer to Part 3, Chapter 2, on Bi Syndromes for more information on this.

Approach

Wherever the muscle spasm is occurring, use local points to get the Qi moving in that specific muscle in order to relieve the muscle spasm. Resolving Bi Syndromes more fully (Obstruction Syndromes) is covered in Part 3, Chapter 2.

Osteoporosis

Associated Element: Water
Associated Organ: Kidney

Analysis

Bones are the tissue of the Water Element. Osteoporosis is a degenerative condition that shows up in older people. "Degenerative condition" gives us the big clue that Kidney Essence is involved.

Osteoporosis also seems to affect women more than men. Where did women's Essence go that men's did not? Where did your original nutrition come from after conception? To nourish a fertilized egg into a thriving baby requires the gift of the Mother's Essence. To endure the nine months of carrying, nourishing, and birthing a baby, she will likely use up some of her precious Essence.

To produce milk, she will need to use some of her Essence as the basis. The endurance required to care for an infant, a toddler, a child, a teenager, a young adult requires her Essence.

How has she cared for herself? How has she protected, nourished, consolidated her Essence? Answers to these questions will have implications for the state of her bones as she ages.

Approach

Prevention is always the best "treatment" for degenerative conditions. Supporting clients to nourish and care for themselves will go a long way in preventing many conditions.

Meridian Massage is not going to reverse osteoporosis, but it may play a role in slowing its progression. Use points to nourish the Kidneys such as KD-3, KD-6, BL-23. If the spine is particularly affected, use SI-3 combined with BL-62 (a Master Point combination), as well as the entire Bladder meridian.

The main role Meridian Massage can play is in helping your clients identify how to better nourish themselves. Use your knowledge of Yin, Yang, and the Five Elements and collaborate with your clients to devise lifestyle adjustments that will help preserve their Essence. Introspection, developing the ability to feel and respond to the needs and desires of our inner world, can be facilitated with thoughtful and skilled massage. In particular, abdominal massage is a powerful tool for awakening to our patterns of habit that do not support our self-care.

Parkinson's Disease

Same as for Alzheimer's Disease.

Plantar Fasciitis

Associated Element: Wood
Associated Organ: Liver

Analysis

The tissue of the Wood Element is the sinews, the tendons, ligaments, and the fibrous connective tissues. Plantar fasciitis points to restriction, stagnation, and dryness in the Wood Element.

The Liver is responsible to maintain the smooth flow of Qi, and for moistening the sinews. The Liver plays a large role in the maintenance of Blood, and in the movement of Blood since Qi is the Commander of Blood. Lack of lubrication of the sinews results in stiffness, loss of elasticity, and constriction of the sinews.

Approach

In addition to local massage, offer support to the Liver in general. As previously discussed, the Liver is overtaxed by modern society's over-emphasis on the Wood Element. Support your clients to access the balancing potential of the Metal Element through increased self-awareness and self-sensitivity as you massage their abdomen and coach them to feel their breath.

GB-34 is the Influential Point (Influential Points are a category of points) for tendons and ligaments, and should be added to your massage. Use LV-3 and BL-18 to soothe and support the Liver.

Respiratory Infections

(Cold, flu, bronchitis, pneumonia, sinusitis, stuffy nose, cough)

Associated Element: Metal
Associated Organ: Lung

Analysis

Respiratory infections are all situated in the Lung Organ system. We have a layer of Qi that defends and protects us—it is called the Wei Qi, or Defensive Qi. The Lung is in charge of keeping the Defensive Qi strong and flowing. The Defensive Qi protects us from external pathogens such as Wind, Cold, Damp, Heat, and Dryness. Western science would add in microbes such as viruses and bacteria.

As mentioned earlier, I refer to the Defensive Qi as my "Qi jacket." As long as we have our Qi jacket on, and it is thick enough and zipped up, external pathogens cannot get into our meridian system.

Approach

Prevention is key here, and supporting the Lung Organ system is the key to our prevention system. As part of the Metal Element, the Lung appreciates quiet, inward time, rest, and reflection. The Lungs are vulnerable to Cold and Dryness which are the climates of the Fall season. Protect the Lung system by staying warm.

Bundle up and wear a scarf to protect yourself from Wind and Cold. Eat warm, moist foods (soup is perfect) in the Fall to support and nourish the Lungs.

Points to nourish the Lungs include LU-1, LU-2, LU-7, and BL-13.

Once any respiratory condition is contracted, rest, warm foods, and quiet are essential parts of the healing process. After the condition is resolved, get to work boosting the Lung system in order to prevent further recurrences.

Notice that respiratory conditions peak in the Fall, which is the season of the Metal Element. If a person is constantly catching colds and flus, it is a clear sign that they need to attend to the Metal Element more consciously throughout the year. Concentrated attention and nourishment of the Metal Element will enable the Lung to maintain a strong Qi jacket, which results in prevention of respiratory illnesses.

During a cold or flu, use the Large Intestine (Yang partner of the Lung) points to clear away the pathogens: LI-4 for headaches, cough, to clear congestion; LI-20 to open the nose; LI-11 to relieve fever. LU-10 is used to relieve sore throat.

Sciatica

Associated Element: Wood
Associated Organs: Gallbladder, Bladder

Analysis

In Western terms, this condition arises from irritation of the sciatic nerve due to impingement somewhere along the length of the nerve. The greater the impingement, the more intense the pain is.

As this is a peripheral nerve syndrome, the Wood Element is in play. The point in the hip where the pain is often focused is usually right at the GB-30 point (see diagram, p. 138). The referred pain travels down either the Gallbladder meridian or the Bladder meridian.

The Liver and Gallbladder are in charge of maintaining the smooth flow of Qi. The main pathology of the Gallbladder meridian is Qi stagnation. Where the Qi stagnates, pain arises. The bigger and more chronic the stagnation, the worse the pain is.

Approach

Physically getting the Qi moving is the treatment for resolving the pain. Preventing recurrence requires resolving Wood-related issues (see "Wood, Element" page 44).

Massage to the Gallbladder meridian from GB-30 all the way to its final point on the fourth toe is helpful. If the pain is traveling along the Bladder meridian, massage that whole meridian to its end point on the pinky toe. Bring movement (not pain) to GB-30. Keep the Qi moving down the Gallbladder meridian using GB-31, 32, 33, 34, 40, 41, and 44. Get the Qi moving down the Bladder meridian using BL-40, 55, 56, 57, 60, and 67.

Spinal issues
(Scoliosis, Kyphosis, Lordosis, C-Curve)

Associated Element: Water
Associated Organ: Kidney

Analysis

As these are conditions of the bones, they all are in the domain of the Water Element, and more specifically the Kidney. The Kidneys hold the Life Force and are responsible for growth, development, and reproduction. Just as congenital issues in Western medicine point to genetics, these same conditions in Chinese medicine point to the Life Force, Essence, to the Kidneys.

Certain spinal conditions are congenital, however, some develop over time with age and degeneration. In both cases the Kidneys are involved.

The Bladder meridian runs parallel to both sides of the spine. Utilize the entire length of the Bladder meridian and local Bladder points to alleviate pain and muscle tension along the spine. Use the Master Point combination of SI-3 + BL-62 to enliven the spine and relieve pain. For details on Master Points see Part 2, Chapter 6.

Meridian Massage alone will not resolve these issues. As with all conditions, there is a need for the client to be very involved in actively moving toward balance. However, Meridian Massage is a reliable method for relieving pain and muscle tension related to these spinal conditions.

TMJ—Temporomandibular Joint Syndrome

Associated Element: Wood
Associated Organ: Gallbladder

Analysis

Clenching the jaw is often done as part of an effort to hold in anger and frustration.

Any tension pattern that holds back any emotion creates a block in the flow of Qi. These patterns are often developed early in life, prior to our conscious awareness of what we are doing. If the pattern continues as we progress through life, it may become so severe that the underlying Qi flow becomes so disrupted that physical manifestations begin to arise.

One-sided complaints are in the territory of the Gallbladder meridian. TMJ often creates pain at one side of the jaw. Ask more questions, and it is likely that your client also suffers from one-sided headaches and sciatic pain on the same side as the TMJ pain.

The Gallbladder meridian traverses the side of the body (see diagram, p. 138). The GB meridian is often the site of Qi stagnation due to its association with the Wood Element. Tight tendons, restricted joint motion due to tight tendons and ligaments—all are in the domain of the Wood Element.

Approach

In the case of TMJ syndrome, the Wood Element must be addressed. In particular, notice how the GB meridian covers the temporalis muscle (located on the sides of the head) and GB-2, GB-3, and ST-7 are very close to the temporomandibular joint.

The treatment intention is simple: Move the Qi. As the practitioner, you can get the Qi moving relatively simply. To resolve the issue, the internal energetic blocks have to be resolved. Like untying a knot of yarn, we untie these energetic knots with patience and loose, open motions. If we pull the strand too tightly, it just creates a tighter knot.

The client's internal awareness is key to this process. The client must address the tension pattern and the energetic, emotional knot that keeps giving rise to the physical manifestation of jaw clenching and teeth grinding. Resolving these energetics results in the alleviation of symptoms all along the meridian.

Tendonitis

Associated Element: Wood
Associated Organs: Liver, Gallbladder

Analysis

The tendons are governed by the Wood Element and therefore by the Liver and Gallbladder, the Organs that maintain the Yin-Yang balance of the Wood Element. For any injury to the tendons, we must look into how the balance of the Liver and Gallbladder is operating.

Acute tendon inflammation will be hot, red, and painful. Chronic tendonitis may be less inflamed, but still painful to the touch.

Acute tendonitis is often an effect of overuse of tendons that are not warmed up, or are asked to work too hard and/or too quickly. Chronic tendonitis is often the result of repetitive motions. In many cases people feel the pain or restriction and override that message in order to continue the repetitive motion.

Wood energy at an extreme is aggressive and competitive. This is a great quality for an Olympic or professional athlete. However, when anyone—professional athlete, weekend warrior, manual laborer, or time-pressured caregiver—ignores pain signals, trouble is on the way.

Approach

There are many effective ways of soothing tendonitis in the short term. For long-term resolution and prevention of continued injury, the Wood energy has to be calmed and the behavior of ignoring pain has to be changed to one of listening and responding. This is a tall order for the ambitious, aggressive, competitive, physically proficient Wood Element. For more on soothing the Wood Element refer to p. 44. For more about the Liver Organ System, refer to the Liver Organ System (pp. 58–60).

As mentioned above, GB-34 is the Influential Point for tendons and ligaments. Regardless of whether the condition is acute or chronic, or the location of the tendonitis, use GB-34. GB-34 is also used preventatively to strengthen the tendons.

Tight Muscles

Associated Elements: Wood, Earth
Associated Organs: Liver, Spleen

Analysis

Muscles require Qi and Blood. When the flow of these is restricted, the muscles become tight. Bi Syndromes can block the flow of Qi and Blood, further complicating the issue. See Part 3, Chapter 2 for information about Bi Syndromes.

Tendons are the tissue of the Liver (Wood) and muscles are the tissue of the Spleen (Earth). Tight tendons arise from Liver Qi stagnation and/or inadequate nourishment from Blood. Circulation of Qi and Blood is supported by physical movement, so sedentary lifestyles are major contributors to this condition.

Issues affecting the muscles are related to the Spleen. The Spleen has a key role in the production of Blood and in sending the Qi and Blood out to the extremities, the muscles.

Approach

Soothe the Liver and support the Spleen. Notice that in the Consolidation Cycle of the Five Elements (see p. 42) the Liver (Wood) consolidates the Spleen (Earth). When the Wood Element is overdeveloped, rather than consolidating the Earth Element it "attacks" the Earth Element. Now we have an over-excited, overtaxed Liver beating up on the Spleen, restricting the Spleen's ability to do its job of absorbing Qi and building Blood. This limitation to the Spleen's function can have a direct impact on the muscles—leading sometimes to muscle fatigue, sometimes to muscle tension and cramping. Soothe the Liver by using LV-3 and BL-18 separately. Support the Spleen using SP-6, ST-36, BL-20, BL-21. The Spleen has everything to do with digestion, so use abdominal massage to support the digestive process, thus helping the weakened Spleen do its job.

Trigger Points

Associated Element: Wood (most often)
Associated Organs: Liver and Gallbladder

Analysis

When Qi stagnates at a point along a meridian, pain is a common symptom. Stagnation along the meridian as it traverses muscles can accumulate and manifest physically as a trigger point. Trigger points are places where Qi can easily stagnate. They often correspond to common acupoints.

Approach

The immediate resolution is to unblock the meridian and get the Qi moving. Stagnations like this are another manifestation of Bi Syndromes (obstruction syndromes). The treatment plan is always the same—open the meridian and get the Qi moving. See Part 3, Chapter 2 for information on Bi Syndromes.

Prevention requires attention to maintaining abundant and flowing Qi in the meridian, preventing exposure to the external pathogens of Cold, Wind, Damp, or Heat.

Ulcerative Colitis

Associated Element: Metal
Associated Organ: Large Intestine

Analysis

Ulcerative colitis is a condition of the Large Intestine, so consider all Metal Element associations. Ulcers and inflammation point to excess heat. This heat needs to be cleared off in conjunction with addressing the Metal Element.

Emotionally, heat can build up from frustration and stagnation associated with the Wood Element. Alcohol, fried foods, red meat, hot and spicy foods all add heat directly into the intestines at the physical level.

Heat, inflammation, and acute flare-ups all point to Yang in excess of Yin. When the energetic imbalance of Yin and Yang becomes more and more extreme, these manifestations also become more extreme. Extreme manifestations require more changes and interventions to resolve.

Approach

Gently approach the large intestine, never cause or exasperate any pain. If there is a current acute flare-up, do not use any deep pressure to the large intestine. The intention is to soothe the Metal Element, so utilize attention to the breath, gentle abdominal massage (unless contra-indicated due to pain and acute episode) to create more room for the movement of the diaphragm.

Use these points to clear heat: LI-11, LI-4, SJ-5, LV-2, GB-34. To nourish the Lungs use LU-1, LU-2, LU-7, LU-9, BL-13. Support the digestion using ST-36, ST-25, SP-15.

In addition to the work on the massage table, the client must make lifestyle changes to reduce the heat and stagnation in their life. When the excess heat clears off and the Qi is again flowing smoothly through the meridian system, the manifestations will also clear up.

2: Conditions by Element

This section reviews some common conditions encountered in a massage therapy practice. To apply the foundational theory in our hands-on work with these and other conditions, we need to evaluate them within the framework of Chinese medicine. The intention of this chapter is to support your understanding of common conditions from the Five Element perspective.

By knowing the Element that is associated with certain conditions you will be able to:

1. Have a beginning framework for which meridians and points to use during the session.

2. Have a beginning framework for which organ(s) to focus on during the abdominal massage portion of the session.

3. Offer your client lifestyle adjustments based on the qualities of the Element that will help balance their system.

I have grouped Conditions by Element to offer you a broad way of approaching these issues and understanding the Elements even more. For each Element I list Conditions that directly affect the organ ("organ" refers here to the Western perspective, meaning the physical organ itself), and Related Conditions. Related Conditions reference the broader perspective of the Organ system from Chinese medicine.

For instance, with the Metal Element there are Conditions that affect the lungs—such as cough and cold—and Related Conditions such as depression and isolation.

Metal

Associated Yin Organ: Lung
Associated Yang Organ: Large Intestine

Conditions affecting the Lungs:

Respiratory conditions—colds, flus, pneumonia, bronchitis, sinusitis, coughs
Allergies
Asthma

Conditions affecting the Large Intestine:

Constipation
Diarrhea
IBS—Irritable bowel syndrome
Ulcerative colitis

Metal Qualities:

Fall
Dry
White
Skin
Nose, smelling
Grief
Letting go
Down, drawn inward, sunken
Courage to move on
Feeling the self
Breathing
Breath

Related Conditions:

Depression
Fatigue
Isolation
"Stuck" in grief

The Metal Element is often neglected in Western cultures. In general, Western cultures do not value processes associated with the Metal Element: going inward, being quiet, meditation, contemplation, reflection, moderation, etc. It can be challenging for us as individuals to bring these practices into our lives in ways that balance a cultural disposition to overdevelop the Wood Element.

The effects of overdeveloping the Wood Element in relation to the Metal Element are easy to see: We often hear that people "don't have time" to meditate, go for a walk, or commit to that yoga class, for example—even though they "really want to." Metal gives us the ability to literally feel ourselves. To feel ourselves, our attention must go inward, the exact opposite of the outward movement of Wood. Wood is Spring, Metal is Fall.

Meridian Massage offers healing to people and to a culture currently caught in an extreme expression of the Wood Element. Creating a quiet, peaceful, tranquil space for individuals to feel themselves, rest, and breathe is itself a remedy to an outsized Wood Element. Teaching people to bring their attention inward, feel themselves, and respond to what they feel offers a process of living that helps individuals take responsibility for their own health and happiness.

Wood

Associated Yin Organ: Liver
Associated Yang Organ: Gallbladder

Conditions affecting the Liver:
Effects of medications, drugs, alcohol on the liver
Liver toxicity
Hepatitis
Cirrhosis

Conditions affecting the Gallbladder:
Gall stones

Wood Qualities:
Spring
Birth
Expansion, ambition, assertion, aggression, anger, protection
Vision
Eyes
Nervous system, fight-or-flight responses
Tendons, ligaments, the "sinews"
Green
Wind

Related Conditions:

Any tendon or ligament injury whether chronic or acute, e,g,, Carpal Tunnel Syndrome, frozen shoulder, Plantar fasciitis, sprained ankle, etc.

Eye issues—blurred vision, floaters, cataracts

Headaches, including migraines

High blood pressure

Menstrual cramps

PMS (Premenstrual Syndrome)

Sciatica

Short temper

Stroke

TMJ (Temporal Mandibular Joint) Syndrome

Overdevelopment of the Wood Element stresses the Liver. When the Liver is overloaded with toxicity from food, air, drugs, and/or emotions, it becomes hot and irritated. This condition manifests as a hot-tempered, angry, impatient, tense person who is over-extended in their responsibilities. Physically they suffer from stiff tendons, tight muscles, high blood pressure, sciatica, headaches, jaw tension, tight neck and shoulders, pain in the area of the liver. They have a difficult time relaxing, going inward, feeling and nourishing themselves.

Meridian Massage offers relief for the excessive Wood qualities that tend to create stagnation in the meridians resulting in many of the conditions listed above. Using meridians and points, the practitioner can support the unblocking of the meridians and the return to a more balanced flow of Qi throughout the entire system. As these blocks are released, relief is experienced in the entire web of the Liver-Gallbladder Organ system, meaning there is a return to balance in the ligaments, tendons, nervous system, emotions, mind, and spirit.

We offer our clients simple and effective lifestyle adjustments so that they can play an active role in their stress reduction without having to change all of their external circumstances. Encouraging a daily walk supports the movement and expansion of Qi that the Wood Element seeks. Teaching clients to feel their breath for even three to five minutes a day brings in the balancing effects of the Metal Element.

By knowing the associations of each of the Five Elements you are able to offer simple tips that really do have a big impact.

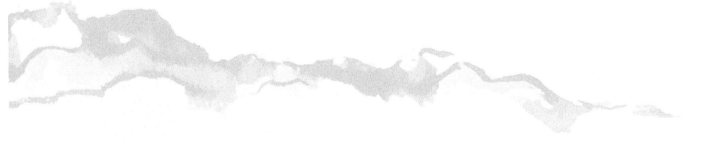

Fire

Associated Yin Organs: Heart, Pericardium
Associated Yang Organs: Small Intestine, San Jiao

Conditions affecting the Heart:

Any cardiac condition
Circulatory issues

Conditions affecting the Pericardium:

Any cardiac condition

Conditions affecting the Small Intestine:

Celiac Disease
Chrohn's Disease
Irritable Bowel Syndrome
Peptic Ulcer

Conditions affecting the San Jiao:

Generalized heat patterns in any of the three burners: the chest cavity, the middle abdomen, the lower abdomen.

Fire Qualities:

Heat, warmth
Red
Tongue
Speech, language, talking
Passions, desires
Love, joy, or the absence of these
If anger is brewing in Wood, it can peak as rage and hatred in Fire.
Communication
Summer
Bright
Extroversion
Control (as the Emperor in charge of everyone).

Related conditions:

Anxiety
Emotional / psychological / psychiatric issues
Heat, inflammation, acute onset
Hyperactivity
Insomnia
Temperature complaints—too hot, or too cold

The Fire Element is often over-emphasized in modern Western culture. There is a cultural bias that it is good to be in control, to be the "big shot," to be social, to talk, to express, to "show off," to be extroverted, to go-go-go and party all night long. This lifestyle often leads to an excessive expression of the Fire Element that over time leads to imbalance.

When the Fire is too big for the Water to balance, it burns "out of control." The extra Fire creates excess heat that can dry up the Water. As the Water continues to diminish, the Fire is even less contained.

The "fuel" of Yang (Fire) is Yin (Water). As the Fire burns off the Water, the Yang literally burns up its fuel source and will eventually go out either abruptly or gradually. Abrupt manifestations may be stroke, heart attack, or a psychotic event.

Meridian Massage brings balance to the whole system, supporting the expression of all Five Elements. As we support our clients to access the resources of all of the Elements, we reduce the habit of exclusively calling up the qualities of the Fire Element to meet every life situation.

For instance, a CEO of a big company will have greater longevity, less stress, and a more versatile staff by delegating authority. When the "big shot" is quiet and listens to others, true communication is possible. Those being listened to by a vibrant and loving person will experience the warmth and inspiration of that person. The benefit for the big Fire personality is that they are able to conserve their energy, quiet their hearts, and enjoy the resources of their Water, Earth, Wood, and Metal Elements.

Water

Associated Yin Organ: Kidney
Associated Yang Organ: Bladder

Conditions affecting the Kidney:
Kidney infection
Kidney stones
Conditions affecting the Bladder
Bladder infection
Urinary tract infection

Water Qualities:
Winter, cold

Ears, hearing

Life Force, Essence (Jing)

Creativity

Sexual energy

Sexual organs

Fertility

Bones, marrow (brain and bone marrow)

Black / Blue

Receptive, still, middle of the night, dark, quiet

Incubating

Longevity, aging

Related Conditions:

ALS

Alzheimer's Disease

Degenerative bone conditions

Dementia

Developmental challenges

Disc herniation, degeneration

Exhaustion

Fertility

Hearing loss

Impotence

Menopausal complaints

Osteoporosis

Parkinson's Disease

Pregnancy

Spine conditions such as scoliosis, lordosis, kyphosis

The Kidneys are associated with the Water Element. They hold the Life Force and govern growth, reproduction, and development—which is why there are so many conditions related to the Water Element.

Meridian Massage is a great way to support and nourish the Water Element. Often the Water Element is exhausted from the fast pace of modern culture and its emphasis on the Fire and Wood Elements. Slowing down and taking time to consciously rest during a massage replenishes the Water Element.

Winter, the season of the Water Element, is a time of incubation and stillness from which infinite possibilities may emerge in Spring. Prior to expression of anything is the time of quiet, of nothing—"no thing," non-expression. By supporting your client to honor their times of incubation you help them nourish and consolidate the valuable resource of their Life Force.

Earth

Associated Yin Organ: Spleen
Associated Yang Organ: Stomach

Conditions affecting the Spleen (and pancreas):
Diabetes
Hypo / hyperglycemia

Conditions affecting the Stomach:
Acid indigestion
Digestion problems
Ulcers

Earth Qualities:
Late Summer
Humid, Damp
The transitions between seasons
Center, middle
Muscles
Presence
Manifestation
Satisfaction, content, abundance, sharing
Give and take
Mothering, nurturing, feeding, eating
Worrying
Mouth and lips
Grounded, security, safety

Related Conditions:
Eating disorders
Gum disease
Fatigue
Fibromyalgia
Muscle weakness
Tooth abscess

Abdominal massage directly affects the Earth Element as we are contacting our client's very center. Working in the abdomen, we help our clients bring their awareness to their center and connect with the Earth Element.

The over-stimulated mind is easily led away from the center, which can contribute to poor choices for the individual. For instance, if one cannot be clear and confident within themselves, they may be swayed to engage in activities that they actually do not want to participate in. This can lead to a cycle of self-doubt and over-reliance on others to make small and large choices for one's life.

Meridian Massage supports self-awareness and self-knowledge through the combination of abdominal massage, meridians, points, and lifestyle adjustments that support the balance of body-mind-spirit. The process of coming to know oneself from the inside out is a hallmark of the Meridian Massage approach, which directly supports the strength, presence, and "centeredness" of the Earth Element.

Part 5

Living Principles: Caring for Yourself to Care for Others

1: Caring for Yourself

It was a particularly challenging time: My Mother was beginning her process of dying. She had just been admitted to hospice. I was bereft, to put it mildly.

As I started to sort my options of going to care for her versus maintaining my commitments—to students, clients, my partner, and myself—a dear friend and healer wrote me in an email:

"It is an act of love for both of you not to forget that the heart pumps blood to itself first."

Walking in the woods another day, pondering how to balance caring for myself and giving love out to others, I heard the message:

"You can only give a glass of water to a thirsty person if you have a glass of water to give them."

These two sentences offer all the guidance I need when considering my own self-care.

We can pretend to give others what we ourselves do not have, but in time everyone will see what is lacking. The practitioner will burn out, feeling that life is unsatisfactory, frustrating, stressful. Clients will feel unsupported, dissatisfied, and go elsewhere for their care.

Each one of us is called to serve others in different ways, for different purposes. Each one of us must wrestle with our own personal growth to develop professionally and feel a sense of wonder, joy, contentment, and interest in our life path. We have to learn how caring for others can actually serve our own aliveness rather than drain us. When we connect to our work from this deeper place, the "work" becomes a joyful extension of our own everyday life.

Most socialization teaches that compassion means thinking of others before thinking of ourselves. In real practice, though, living that way all the time results in resentment and/or a very drained person in need of filling up by others. To truly love another person, to truly give attention, patience, compassion, and time to an other, we must first be able to provide all these things to ourselves. Then we will actually have that glass of water to give another person and not go thirsty ourselves.

To guide clients toward their deepest selves and their own self-awareness, we must travel that path ourselves. This is called walking our talk. You can't be a person of honesty and integrity and ask someone else to live up to ideals that you haven't been able to achieve yourself. Without integrity, your words and your work are empty and your clients will not progress. With integrity and honesty, your words and your work are full of Qi, and your clients will progress.

To have integrity, we must walk our talk. If we find that we are unable to do so, then perhaps we need to temper our talk, make it a more real and better reflection of our truth. This doesn't mean lowering standards, it means being honest with where you are on the path. It means being no more and no less than all that you are, and trusting that will be enough.

If you take the time to care for yourself, you will have the energy and the ability to connect with your Qi, and through that to the Mysterious Source of Nature, the source of everyone's Qi. You will become a clear channel for that Source Qi to flow through, and you will be of true benefit to yourself and your clients.

There is no fooling the Source Qi. You either are in connection with it or you are not. You will be able to feel and know the quality of your connection with Source Qi as long as you persevere with your inward journey.

A lack of self-nourishment is the basis of many illnesses. For that reason, you must be able to offer clear guidance to the self-nourishing ability in your clients. As long as you have taken up and are attending to that task yourself, you will be able to help them do the same.

When you travel the path of self-nourishment, you will be healthier and happier yourself. From that foundation you will be able to offer others a level of healing that is beyond the usual experience of relieving symptoms.

Caring for ourselves can seem like an easy thing to do. But if it were, there would not be so much need and resentment in so many people. This caring is a very simple principle, one you have practiced many times. You find a cup, you go to the faucet, you turn on the water, fill the cup, and place it in the hands of the asker. Your task is done. Drinking the water is up to the other person.

Now make this external practice your inner work. Transform this metaphor into your healing practice.

You feel your body, you follow your breath, you bring your attention inward, you connect to Source Qi, you open yourself to the flow of Source Qi, you put your hands on the other person and allow that Source Qi to connect with their meridian system. You are, in essence, the faucet. The credit you take is for the effort you make to be a clear, willing channel for this flow. Nothing more, and nothing less.

Simple. Not easy. Worth every moment of effort.

2: Self-Care Practices

There is no one way to care for yourself. We each find our own practices that serve us. Here are a few suggestions to get you started. Give them a try, notice what works best, and do more of that.

1. Walking. Simply taking a walk at least once a day brings many benefits. We move our joints in a gentle manner, get our blood and Qi moving, release stagnant Qi and air from our lungs, and have time to contemplate. I suggest walking at least twenty minutes, alone, without talking on the phone or listening to music. The reason to be alone and away from extraneous auditory input is to give your senses and mind time to settle and clear from all of the input they are exposed to throughout the day.

2. Gentle movement or stretching. Move every joint and gently stretch and open the joints. You may be drawn to a particular type of physical activity, such as Qi Gong, Yoga, Zumba, Pilates, etc.—be sure to make time for these practices that support the vitality of your physical structure.

3. Interest or hobby. Make time to pursue an interest or hobby that you enjoy. This serves your Spirit. Attending to the call of our Spirit brings us the richness and meaning of our life. When we express our Spirit we are living the life of our dreams, rather than dreaming of the life that we hope might one day "happen" for us.

3: Following Your Way

The Tao is often referred to as "The Way" when translated into English. The undifferentiated Source Qi, the Wu Qi, the Source, the Divine, Mysterious Source of Nature—these terms all refer to the Tao.

Again, from the Tao Te Ching

The Tao that can be told is not the eternal Tao.
The name that can be named is not the eternal name.
The nameless is the beginning of heaven and earth.
The named is the mother of the ten thousand things.
Ever desireless, one can see the mystery.
Ever desiring, one sees the manifestations.
These two spring from the same source but differ in name:
this appears as darkness.
Darkness within darkness.
The gate to all mystery. [30]

The Tao calls us to be natural, to go with the flow, to be in our flow, to not work so hard at doing but to put our attention, our effort, into Being. Meridian Massage is an approach to bodywork that seeks to utilize the flow of the Tao in service to healing. The meridians and Qi flowing in them offer the most direct physical connection to this Source energy in the body.

There are definite pathways and points to be understood so that our contact is precise and thoughtful. Our confident and correct understanding of the anatomical locations of the meridians supports our ability to simply be present in a particular moment with a particular person, and trust the flow of Qi that is coming to us and through us, for the benefit of the other.

One person can share only the results of their own experience with another person. We cannot give our experience away or force it upon another. A method can be offered, a door opened, a meeting point arranged, but it always depends upon the seeker, the student, to take up the practices. In taking them up, we step onto a path taken by many others, yet it has no obvious directions, signposts, or finish lines. Each person must find their own way. The only established direction given by the sages through time is to go within, find your own way, and be true to yourself.

Every practitioner of Meridian Massage will have unique techniques and methods that emerge from their inner connection to Nature. The common ground is exploring the value of harmonizing Qi. This requires a leap of faith, followed by thoughtful practice and reflection on one's experience.

Only one who has explored this avenue for themselves and found it to be a match to their experience can offer such a possibility to another. Qi is difficult to comprehend. We find our peace, health, and solace when we are aligned with Nature in such a way that our Qi remains ever flowing toward balance and harmony.

The Tao that can be named is not the Tao. No one can tell you what it is. No one can give it to you. It is freely available to everyone. Each person must take their own turn inward and realize Tao for themselves. Every path is unique, every expression unique.

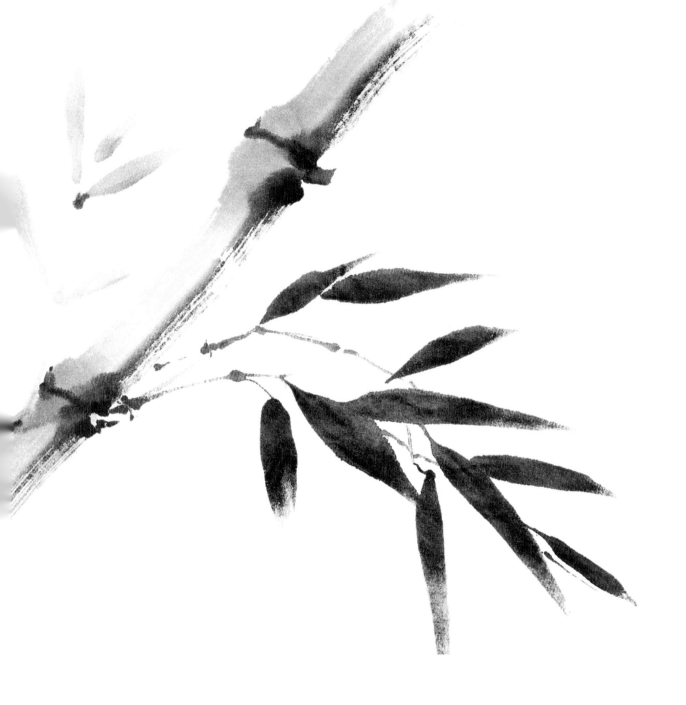

May your journey be ever
adventurous and joyful!

Points Contra-indicated in Pregnancy

- All deep massage on abdomen
- All points on the abdomen
- GB-21
- LI-4
- SP-6
- KD-1
- BL 31–34
- UB-60
- UB-67 —this is traditionally used to turn the fetus at the end of term if it is in a breach position.

The logic behind these contra-indicated points and areas:

One challenge of pregnancy is holding the fetus within the uterus. In order to do this we must have plenty of Qi to support holding the fetus up and in against the contrast of gravity's downward pull.

The points that naturally draw the Qi downward are contra-indicated in pregnancy.
These same points will be of benefit during labor and delivery.

Deep massage to the abdomen is contra-indicated to protect the fetus.

Point Index

NUMBER	PINYIN	ENGLISH
LU-1	Zhong Fu	Middle Palace
LU-2	Yun Men	Cloud Gate
LU-5	Chi Ze	Cubit Marsh
LU-7	Lie Que	Broken Sequence
LU-9	Tai Yuan	Great Abyss
LU-10	Yu Ji	Fish Border
LI-4	He Gu	Joining Valley
LI-10	Shou San Li	Arm Three Miles
LI-11	Qu Chi	Pool at the Crook
LI-20	Ying Xiang	Welcome Fragrance
ST-2	Si Bai	Four Whites
ST-5	Da Ying	Great Welcome
ST-6	Jia Che	Jaw Bone
ST-7	Xia Guan	Below the Joint
ST-12	Que Pen	Empty Basin
ST-25	Tian Shu	Heavens's Pivot
ST-34	Liang Qiu	Ridge Mound
ST-36	Zu San Li	Leg Three Miles
ST-41	Jie Xi	Stream Divide
ST-44	Nei Ting	Inner Courtyard
SP-4	Gong Sun	Grandfather Grandson
SP-6	San Yin Jiao	Three Yin Meeting
SP-8	Di Ji	Earth Pivot
SP-9	Yin Ling Quan	Yin Mound Spring
SP-10	Xue Hai	Sea of Blood
SP-15	Da Heng	Great Horizontal
HT-3	Shao Hai	Lesser Sea
HT-5	Tong Li	Penetrating the Interior
HT-7	Shen Men	Spirit Gate
SI-3	Hou Xi	Back Stream
SI-9	Jian Zhen	True Shoulder
SI-10	Nao Shu	Upper Arm Shu
SI-18	Quan Liao	Cheek Bone Crevice
SI-19	Ting Gong	Palace of Hearing
BL-10	Tian Zhu	Celestial Pillar

NUMBER	PINYIN	ENGLISH
BL-13	Fei Shu	Lung Shu
BL-14	Jue Yin Shu	Pericardium Shu
BL-15	Xin Shu	Heart Shu
BL-18	Gan Shu	Liver Shu
BL-19	Dan Shu	Gallbladder Shu
BL-20	Pi Shu	Spleen Shu
BL-21	Wei Shu	Stomach Shu
BL-22	San Jiao Shu	San Jiao Shu
BL-23	Shen Shu	Kidney Shu
BL-25	Da Chang Shu	Large Intestine Shu
BL-27	Xiao Chang Shu	Small Intestine Shu
BL-28	Pang Guan Shu	Bladder Shu
BL-31	Shang Liao	Upper Crevice
BL-32	Ci Liao	Second Crevice
BL-33	Zhong Liao	Middle Crevice
BL-34	Xia Liao	Lower Crevice
BL-36	Cheng Fu	Hold and Support
BL-40	Wei Zhong	Middle of the Crook
BL-55	He Yang	Confluence of Yang
BL-56	Cheng Jin	Support the Sinews
BL-57	Cheng Shan	Support the Mountain
BL-60	Kun Lun	Kunlun Mountains
BL-62	Shen Mai	Extending Vessel
BL-67	Zhi Yin	Reaching Yin
KD-1	Yong Quan	Bubbling Spring
KD-2	Ran Gu	Blazing Valley
KD-3	Tai Xi	Supreme Stream
KD-6	Zhao Hai	Shining Sea
KD-10	Yin Gu	Yin Valley
KD-22	Bu Lang	Walking Corridor
KD-23	Shen Feng	Spirit Seal
KD-24	Ling Xu	Spirit Ruins
KD-25	Shen Cang	Spirit Storehouse
KD-26	Yu Zhong	Comfortable Chest
KD-27	Shu Fu	Shu Mansion
P-6	Nei Guan	Inner Gate
P-7	Da Ling	Great Mound
P-8	Lao Gong	Palace of Toil

NUMBER	PINYIN	ENGLISH
SJ-3	Zhong Zhu	Central Islet
SJ-5	Wai Guan	Outer Gate
SJ-21	Er Men	Ear Gate
GB-1	Tong Zi Liao	Pupil Crevice
GB-2	Ting Hui	Meeting of Hearing
GB-12	Wan Gu	Mastoid Process
GB-14	Yang Bai	Yang White
GB-20	Feng Chi	Wind Pool
GB-21	Jian Jing	Shoulder Well
GB-25	Jing Men	Capital Gate
GB-26	Dai Mai	Belt Vessel
GB-30	Huan Tiao	Jumping Circle
GB-31	Feng Shi	Wind Market
GB-32	Zhong Du	Middle Ditch
GB-33	Xi Yang Guan	Knee Yang Gate
GB-34	Yang Ling Quan	Yang Mound Spring
GB-40	Qiu Xu	Mound of Ruins
GB-41	Zu Lin Qi	Foot Governor of Tears
LV-2	Xing Jian	Moving Between
LV-3	Tai Chong	Great Rushing
LV-8	Qu Quan	Spring at the Crook
Du-1	Chang Qiang	Long Strong
Du-4	Ming Men	Life Gate
Du-16	Feng Fu	Palace of Wind
Du-20	Bai Hui	Hundred Meetings
Ren-1	Hui Yin	Meeting of Yin
Ren-4	Guan Yuan	Gate of Origin
Ren-6	Qi Hai	Sea of Qi
Ren-12	Zhong Wan	Middle Cavity
Ren-17	Shan Zhong	Chest Center

Notes

1. Gia-Fu Feng and Jane English, trans., Tao Te Ching (New York: Vintage, 1989), 3

2. Feng and English, Tao Te Ching, editors' note, 87–88

3. Feng and English, Tao Te Ching, 3

4. Feng and English, Tao Te Ching, 3

5. Carl Sagan, Cosmos: A Personal Voyage

6. Maoshing Ni, The Yellow Emperor's Classic of Medicine: A New Translation of the Neijing Suwen with Commentary (Boston: Shambhala, 1995), 53

7. Feng and English, Tao Te Ching, editors' commentary, 87–88,

8. Feng and English, Tao Te Ching, 3

9. Feng and English, Tao Te Ching, 27

10. Peter Deadman and Mazin Al-Khafaji, with Kevin Baker, A Manual of Acupuncture (East Sussex, England: Journal of Chinese Medicine Publications, 2006), 11 (quoting Ling Shu or The Spiritual Pivot, Chapter 17)

11. Feng and English, Tao Te Ching, 10

12. For information on Command Points, see Part 2, Chapter 7.

13. See Chapter 6 here in Part 2 for information on Master Points.

14. I discuss Ren in Chapter 2 of Part 2.

15. See Part 2, Chapter 5.

16. See Part 2, Chapter 6.

17. See Part 2, Chapter 4 for information on Yuan Source Points.

18. See Part 2, Chapter 2 for information on extraordinary vessels.

19. Meaning "Greatest Yang." The Bladder meridian is the most external meridian (in Six Channel Theory) and so is often the first meridian to be invaded by external pathogens.

20. See Part 2, Chapter 2.

21. See Part 2, Chapter 6.

22. Meaning "Bright Yang."

23. See Part 2, Chapter 6.

24. See Part 2, Chapter 6.

25. See Part 2, Chapter 6.

26. Wu Jing-Nuan trans., Ling Shu or Spiritual Pivot (Washington DC: Taoist Center Press, 2002), 88

27. Feng and English, Tao Te Ching, 47. I have modified the translation slightly, substituting "The sage" for "He" in the last two lines. The Chinese term in the original text is gender neutral.

28. Maoshing Ni, The Yellow Emperor's Classic of Medicine, 11

29. Maoshing Ni, The Yellow Emperor's Classic of Medicine, 7

30. Feng and English, Tao Te Ching, 3

Index

N

O

P

Q

R

S

About the Author

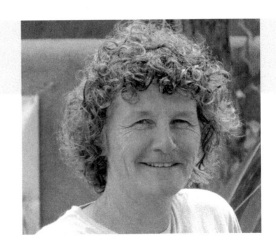

Cindy Black, L.Ac., LMT, is one of about 7.3 billion people on this Earth hoping for a good and meaningful life.

The founder of Big Tree School of Natural Healing, she is an acupuncturist and a massage therapist with more than twenty years' experience as a teacher and hands-on practitioner. She integrates Classical Chinese medicine and Western massage therapy in a unique approach to balancing mind, body, and spirit—a practice known as Meridian Massage.

Her profound thinking, humor, and unique ability to make the complex accessible combine to help these much-needed teachings inspire many people throughout the world.

Study with her at www.bigtreehealing.com.

About the Artist - Jessica Joswiak

The composition of the human body informs everything I do as a visual artist.

The line-work of our bone structure and muscle tissue, along with the complexity of how we function is at the core of my work. I am constantly looking at the sculptures of Manuel Neri, and the drawings of Gustav Klimt, as their expressiveness is so inspiring. I also look to the meticulous details in medical illustrations to inform the technical elements of my drawings.

As a child I was taught the importance of alternative medicine, massage, and energy based healing. So making drawings for this book combined my passion for art with my appreciation of alternative healing methodology, and it's been an absolute honor to be involved in this project.

Study with Cindy

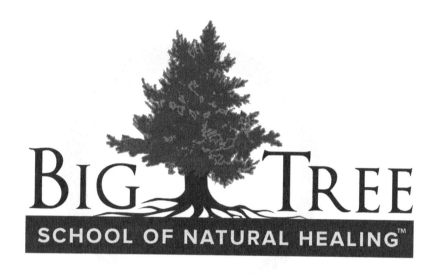

Go to:
www.BigTreeHealing.com

Cindy's Blog:
www.Bigtreehealing.com/blog

Connect on Facebook:
www.facebook.com/bigtreehealing/

CPSIA information can be obtained
at www.ICGtesting.com
Printed in the USA
LVOW01s1721070316

478106LV00028B/62/P

9 780996 971812